RetroAge ®

RetroAge®

THE FOUR-STEP PROGRAM TO REVERSE THE AGING PROCESS

HATTIE
with SALLIE BATSON

FOREWORD BY DR. JOHN KILDAHL

BERKLEY BOOKS, NEW YORK

Before beginning any new diet, nutrition or exercise program, consult with a physician, especially if you have any serious condition or are taking medication. The author and publisher disclaim responsibility for any adverse effects or unforeseen consequences resulting from the use of the information contained in this book.

RETRoAGE®

A Berkley Book / published by arrangement with
the authors

PRINTING HISTORY
Berkley trade paperback edition / February 1997

The Putnam Berkley World Wide Web site address is http://www.berkley.com/berkley

ISBN: 0-425-15611-7

BERKLEY®
Berkley Books are published by The Berkley Publishing Group,
200 Madison Avenue, New York, New York 10016.
BERKLEY and the "B" design
are trademarks belonging to Berkley Publishing Corporation.

PRINTED IN THE UNITED STATES OF AMERICA

10   9   8   7   6   5   4   3   2   1

A percentage of the profits from this book will be given to EarthSave and to PETA (People for the Ethical Treatment of Animals).

All photographs of Hattie appearing in this book have not been retouched.

For my mother, Sarah,
who always knew I would achieve my dreams,
and for my father, Natie,
who was embarrassed that I might . . .

Watch over me.

WITH APPRECIATION...

Without explanation, but with considerable gratitude, I wish to acknowledge Martha Andrews, Lou Bartfield, Jacques Borris, Joel Benjamin, Lisa Berkley, Pat Betty, Portia Bowers, Dale Burg, Pam Burt, Desmond Child, Carrie Coakley, Martin Cohen, Patricia Collins, Dr. Harry Collymore (Trinidad), Andrew Connolly, Chris Connolly, Denise DeBaun, Ben Dolphin, Bernard Dunayevich, Diane Eichenbaum, Dolores Engel, Stephany Evans, Bruce Fenton, Helen and Joe Frett (Tortola), Edna Frome, Elane Geller, Jim Graham, Len Grau, Dr. Gerry Herman, Dr. Steve Hoody, Susan Johann, Laurie Kaufman, Michele and Stanley Kaufman, Dr. John Kildahl, Concepción Lara, Bonnie and Wayne Laszlow, Colin Lively, Chuck London, Joy Pierson, Anastasia Piper, Bart Potenza, Margaretta Richards, Eve Robinson, Laurie and Darren Shields, Roger Smith and Landmark Education Corp., Bonnie Solow, Kelly Walters, Joshua Wiener, Rama Wiener, Michael Wyman and Muhammed Yakub. And Hattie Arnone for heart and hearth. And Sallie Batson, without whom, and more. And Denise Silvestro for her on-target editing and powerful support. And Joni Friedman for the eye of the artist.

CONTENTS

FOREWORD

William Shakespeare saw aging this way: "Pouch on side . . . youthful hose too wide . . . his shrunk shank . . . big manly voice turned to childish treble . . . pipes and whistles in his sound . . . last scene . . . sans teeth, sans eyes, sans taste . . ."

That was four hundred years ago.

Now comes Hattie.

In a book small enough to carry in your bag are ideas enough to fill a healthy lifetime. This is a first-person story, intimately personal. Hattie has been there, done that. Early experiences of seeing her mother's aging body have affected her whole life and, thankfully, have motivated her to design a comprehensive program of RetroAging. Early on, Hattie's own body became her battleground. Readers will feel the self-loathing that she felt about her body. There are painful self-revelations here: feelings that many people have, but which they keep secret, often even to themselves. Hattie won that inner struggle. She won the battle and she vividly tells how others can do it too. Hattie turned the aging clock back through her personal experience and her careful study of aging. Her answer is RetroAge.

Persons long in years are becoming a larger percentage of our population. The life span of the average American increases each year. New questions need new answers. What is aging? What can a person do about it? What about sex drive? What emotional problems do older people have? Does retirement mean regression? When one spouse dies, what can the survivor do to stay alive? And what about recent and remote memory? Can anything be done? Does the brain deteriorate? Do the genes determine your life span? How can the elderly respect themselves and gain the respect of others? How can a fifty-, sixty-, seventy-, eighty-, ninety-, hundred-year-old RetroAge?

Hattie has answers, and she is a communicator. She offers

RetroAging, RetroAge Eating, RetroAge Exercise and Innercize, along with her attitude-shifting Hattietudes. She zings the reader with verbal bullets that penetrate the mind. Again and again, the truth she offers sinks into one's common sense and good judgment.

From my professional vantage point as a clinical psychologist, I looked for what the book offered for the emotional life as well as the physical life. The clearly described programs speak to the quality and quantity of one's life. What warms one's muscles will warm one's mind. An active body allows one to be active socially, intellectually and emotionally.

Aging is in the eye and attitude of the beholder. Genes account for far less than half of how a person adapts to her or his years.

Successful living is in one's motivation and determination. It is also in the skin, arms and legs of the user. Use it or lose it. Hattie shows how to use it and make it better and younger. An active body makes for an active, youthful spirit. Exercise strengthens the bones and the brain. High levels of body stimulation stimulate the intelligence. Some people have begun jogging in their eighties. They have also learned Greek and Sanskrit at the same age. Muscle stretching goes hand in hand with stretching the reach of the brain cells.

"Blitzing" is Hattie's term for taking an active role in one's life, an exciting venture for cleaning out the stuff that ties one to an unhealthy lifestyle. No one wants to sink into a helpless decline. Now we know how not to become feeble.

We all know people who are old at fifty and others who are young at ninety. Some people seem to have little to live for when they pass their twenty-ninth birthday and others feel exhilarated when they become "Senior Citizens." We know persons who have grown in wisdom, seizing the day with an active body and an inquisitive mind.

"Something to do, somewhere to go, someone to love" is a motto that gives meaning to life. A healthy body provides the energy for connecting with friends, neighbors, families, worthy causes. Years bring stories to tell, gifts to share, a perspective worth hearing.

RetroAge offers a breakthrough to the affirmation of life, plus the vitality to enjoy and share it with all humankind.

JOHN P. KILDAHL, PH.D.
Clinical Psychologist/Psychoanalyst
New York, NY

INTRODUCTION

There comes a point in each of our lives that we become inescapably preoccupied with aging.

For some of us, it happens early: When we see those first tiny wrinkles in the corners of our eyes, or when we just can't shed those few extra pounds we packed on over the holidays.

With the passage of years, these early concerns bloom full out, and as we approach our forties, we become actively frightened of becoming old. For many of us, forty is *serious*. It's awfully close to fifty. And very few people can think of fifty as young. Fifty starts sounding like old fogy or, even more dreaded, senior citizen.

I have written this book to bring you to a totally different way of experiencing aging, and to illustrate how this stereotyped negative view dominates reality, finally determining how we actually age. Certainly, it seems we are justified in dreading the aging process. We can look about us and see unattractive older people. We see the diseases, the wheelchairs, the halting gait, the poor memory, sluggishness, sadness, false teeth, nursing homes. It's frightening. Sadly, many people's lives do become awful as they age; however, I assert this happens through negative conditioning.

With RetroAge, you have a choice. Either you can, quite literally, stand by and wait for your face to wrinkle, your joints to ache and your memory to fade, or you can *choose* to take action and reverse almost all negative aspects of aging.

I have never been a timid person—and doing things in moderation never appealed to me. When I found myself beginning to age unattractively, I panicked. I found the slight stoop in my spine and the loss of spring in my step odious. No way was I going to let myself become a decrepit old woman.

I feverishly began to test techniques, personally and professionally, that taught me not only how to age better, but how to actually reverse my aging process. I was relentless.

As a dancer, teacher, therapist and healer, I had long been keenly aware of how my own body worked: which foods lifted my energy and which dragged me down; what made my skin feel soft and smooth, and which exercises made my body supple and strong. I applied this knowledge to my aging, and before long, all the unattractiveness began to disappear. I was astonished at how much better I began to feel. An unexpected bonus from these actions: I not only *felt* younger than my calendar age, I *looked* remarkably younger as well.

When friends and clients wanted to know what I was doing, I willingly shared my secrets with them and learned that my personal age reversal was no fluke. Others who followed my regimen grew younger too.

This might seem like an impossible dream or an empty promise. Granted, some of my ideas may seem peculiar at first, but they have been proven effective time and time again in my private practice and group work.

With RetroAging, you will train yourself to eat healthfully. You will learn ways to improve your skin texture and muscle tone. Your posture, flexibility, strength, endurance and, most importantly, your attitude will be permanently altered.

As you revolutionize your thinking, you will transform the so-called "natural" course of events. Instead of anticipating a long decline, you will experience a shift in consciousness—a shift that transforms aging into an adventure, an opportunity and a gift.

RetroAge teaches you to experience aging as a priceless treasure, the treasure of time. Time in which you can fashion your life to your own specifications.

If you give in and allow nature to take its usual course, in all probability you will age as unattractively as you always feared you would. On the other hand, if you embrace aging as a welcome challenge, you can actually be the architect of your life.

With RetroAge, you create a whole new way of youthful aging that will become the matrix for the rest of your life. This is no quick fix. You will be both the designer and the product. It is a splendid journey. I wish I could assure you the path is easy to follow. It isn't. It takes continual hard work, but you become unstoppable. Why not, when the payoff is so rewarding?

At sixty, my own youthfulness astonishes me. Goals I set at fifty have been surpassed. My energy is boundless. Qualities I once believed were only possessed by the young are once again mine. I say "once again," because I was already "old" when I began my experimentation. My skin was lifeless and dry. I had begun to lose muscle tone and my joints often ached. By the end of a day's work, I was exhausted, and I blamed it on aging. I too had bought into the stereotypical negative image of aging society hands us. I was already choreographing a dirge for my old age.

RetroAge entered my life as a divine gift, at a time when I was feeling old, alone and depressed. As a forty-eight-year-old divorced woman alone in New York City, I was forced to face myself squarely. Initially I was discouraged and felt unattractive and undesirable. Fortunately, I was blessed with the instinct to return to my roots, to once again throw myself into things that I had loved to do as a young woman, activities that had helped make me vibrant and attractive in my youth.

In this book, I share the RetroAge program I discovered with you. You need no special powers to reverse and retard your aging. You do not need to start with enormous drive or self-discipline. Everything you need to age exquisitely is already inside of you. Step by step, your own progress will serve as the inspiration that keeps you going, as it has for me and my clients.

Welcome to this journey.

Hattie

RetroAge®

1 MY VICTORY OVER AGING

IF I CAN DO IT, SO CAN YOU

I refuse to accept society's negative picture of aging. That's the one you and I grew up with. Through my own exploration into ways to maintain youth, I have discovered that the body doesn't know what you want unless you tell it. As soon as you are clear about your needs and expectations and start treating yourself exquisitely, it begins to grow younger. Yes, it's truly possible to age in reverse.

When I was a little girl, my mother would take me along for her weekly visits to the ladies' bathhouse in Brighton Beach.

The women—most of them European émigrés like my mom—relished their time together in the steam room. These ritual sweat baths were social and cleansing, as they chatted and scrubbed away the dirt and tension that clung to their ample bodies.

This was such a treat for my mother that she never realized what a torture it was for me, the only child in the place. Here we were, barely a block from my beloved beach. I longed to be swimming and building sand castles, not sweating with a bunch of old ladies.

The heat and steam that they found so invigorating was suffocating to me. I would crouch toward the floor, gasping for cooler air and dreaming of the frozen custard Mommy would buy for me on our way home.

1

When I looked up, my curious eyes were riveted by the images of the damp, naked bodies towering over me. To this day, I can see them, silhouetted in the acrid steam: lumpy flesh, bellies stretched and flabby, pendulous breasts, purple veins coursing up dimpled legs. This terrified me. "If this is what ladies look like," I innocently vowed, "I don't ever want to be a lady. I'll stay like I am right now."

I could never have imagined then, that now, some fifty-five years later, I would be totally devoted to the human body, loving it in all its forms and imperfections. I had no idea that my childlike revulsion would become my life's passion.

I was a wild child. We lived in a low-income housing project in Williamsburg, Brooklyn, a closely knit community where there was no traffic and plenty of room for me to play safely. Outside my window there was a playground with swings, slides and seesaws. I spent my childhood years a tomboy, running, climbing, playing ball, jumping rope and roller skating . . . until I sprouted breasts. This was a decidedly unwelcome event. Like it or not, I realized, they were there to stay.

It was clear that I was turning into a "lady" despite my best intentions.

My dear mother, an excellent seamstress, made all of my clothes. She used no patterns, instead fashioning garments from fabric remnants which she appliquéd and embroidered beautifully. Sadly, everything she sewed for me was too small, so I always felt as if I had been stuffed into my clothes. Even at this early age my body image was distorted. My body was small and well proportioned, yet I felt too big. Fat.

Because my mother did nothing to maintain or improve the shape of her own body, other than bemoan the fact that she didn't look like the reed-thin models in the high fashion magazines she brought home from the library, I thought that I had no say in how *my* body would look. I inherited my negative self-image from my mom.

I had always been physically active but had no formal dance or art training. There was no money for such luxuries. However, I did show a talent for drawing and painting, so the guidance counselor at my neighborhood junior high school told my parents, "Hattie is special; so she should go to a special school."

Ironically, rather than requesting an application to the High School of Music and Art, which taught the fine arts plus music, my counselor sent for an application to the famed High School for the *Per-*

forming Arts. So, instead of preparing a portfolio of drawings and paintings for the entrance process, I began to work on the two dramatic monologues the instructions ordered. While I had no experience in this sort of thing, I went to work without question. I picked one, the part of a switchboard operator, because I had worked a switchboard on my summer job and related to what this woman was doing. The other monologue was by a woman who had been sentenced to prison. For that, I practiced for hours before the mirror, learning to cry on cue.

There were about five hundred applicants for only fifty or so openings in my class. Miraculously, I was admitted, even though I had no prior drama or dance training. The first dance class I ever took was Movement for Actors, a course in the Drama Department. I took to the stretches and steps as if I had been born moving to music. I was a dancer.

When I danced, my body became truly alive, as when I was a child. I loved how my shapely, teenaged body felt as it moved with the music. It excited me to adorn it, exhibit it, to have it appreciated. But it was one thing to be dancing, the center of a circle of admirers, and quite another to truly experience self-love. Out of class, when I wasn't dancing, these good feelings left me.

Caught up in the beauty of the movement, the music and costumes, I was completely happy, totally distracted from the gnawing discontent that plagued me. Home alone, I continually worried that I could never meet the standards I had set for myself, standards I drew from movies and magazines and from the bone-thin dancers I saw on stage. I soothed my spirit by compulsively eating, which only compounded my problem.

I believed that I could only look pretty fully clothed. I *knew* that concealed beneath my carefully selected wardrobe and confined by my girdle, were what I feared most: flabby thighs, stretch marks, cellulite and a pear-shaped bottom, just like my mother's. Even more horrifying, I perceived varicose veins already forming on my legs.

I was repulsed by my body.

And I was only sixteen.

In retrospect, I acknowledge how distorted these images were. I am five feet, four inches tall, with a finely proportioned, shapely body. At that time, I weighed 122 pounds, seven pounds more than I do right now. I saw myself as huge. In my fantasies, I was five-ten, long-limbed and lean, small-breasted, 110 pounds, with long straight hair. No wonder my self-image suffered. Who I saw in my mirror and who I wanted to see were in no way alike.

This started a lifelong battle to be thin.

One week I downed countless hot fudge sundaes and wore baggy pants; the next, I consumed nothing but grapefruit and black coffee and squeezed into my tightest skirts. My weight went up and down, and so did my moods.

This continued after I entered Brooklyn College, where I became president of the Dance Club. I cultivated my technique and worked on my craft, studying and dancing as much as four hours a day.

This made me even more painfully aware of my body. Others admired my shape and form, but *I* knew what lay jiggling under my leotard and tights. I became obsessed with ridding my body of what I experienced as ugly fat. The cycle of dieting continued.

My talents as a dancer earned me a scholarship to study with the famed Martha Graham, José Limón and Murray Louis at the prestigious Connecticut College School of the Dance, in New London. While there, amid this array of exquisitely toned bodies, I resolved to whip *my* body into shape so I could compete with them. I couldn't be tall, but certainly I could get thin. Besides, I was an outstanding dancer.

And thin I became. I quit eating, except on weekends, when my date—always a cadet from the nearby Coast Guard Academy—took me to the Captain's Table for a lobster dinner. The way I packed it in he certainly had no way of knowing I consumed only a few crackers and water the rest of the week.

My midweek boyfriend, a dashing dancer, Jack Wiener from Detroit, Michigan, never noticed anything was wrong with my eating habits. All female dancers are a little weird about their bodies anyway. Besides, our schedules were so different we never ate our meals together.

I was able to keep my obsession to become rail thin a secret from everyone.

This continued for more than nine months, even after I returned home for my senior year at Brooklyn College.

I went from my healthy, normal weight to a gaunt 108 and looked like a cadaver. I thought I looked sensational. My breasts shrank and my stomach was finally flat, never mind that my menstrual cycle stopped for almost a year. This certainly didn't bother me, but my family was frightened, so my mother carted me off to a gynecologist.

I was anorectic.

The doctor cautioned me that if I kept this up, I might never be able to have children. That was the turning point. All my life I had wanted to be a mother more than anything in the world. I took the little green estrogen pills she gave me and rounded out again.

My breasts and hips returned. It was clear to me that no matter how well I moved or how expressively I danced, I would never look and feel like a *real* dancer—which, to me, meant a super-skinny classical prima ballerina. I surrendered my fantasy of being a performer and became a teacher, a choice I have not once regretted.

Did you think I'd ever give up my dancing? Not on your life. It meant too much to me.

Though I wasn't going to be a performer, I continued to study. And I kept dancing—ballet, flamenco, Israeli and modern dance—and once I had earned my degree from Brooklyn College, I went to teach at Pembroke, the women's college of Brown University. This girl from Brooklyn had made it to the Ivy League!

It was an extraordinary year: I couldn't afford private school and now one was paying me to do something I loved—dance. And since dance was part of the Phys Ed Department, I got to teach swimming and volleyball too.

Did all this athletic activity turn me into a jock? No, it made me ravenous, and gave me justification for eating as much as I wanted. I even hid family packs of Peanut M&Ms in the pockets of my regulation gym suit so that I could munch during volleyball sessions.

Another part of my job was to be housemother in a dorm of about twenty-two freshmen girls. Every night, once I was certain all my charges were present and accounted for, I shut my door and ate bags of sweets in secret. Once again, feelings of inadequacy overtook me. I was a poor girl from the projects. I thought there was no way for me to measure up to the privileged backgrounds of the young women in my care, filled with china and crystal, trust funds and debutante balls. So I ate to make myself feel better.

I hid my anguish so well that I don't think anyone knew how lonely and unhappy I was. After all, I always wore a smile and behaved so cheerfully. It was as if I were two people.

Even though I was proud of my work and had the praise of my students and faculty, my basic self-image remained negative. I stuffed my fears and feelings with food. I wanted to be married and to have a family, yet I was alone, living on the campus of a girls' school, with no prospective husbands in sight. I didn't want to become an old-maid college professor.

I turned to food for solace. I ballooned to a well-rounded 142 pounds on my petite frame. As you can imagine, this was embarrassing to me, since I had to be in a leotard or swimsuit every day. Fortunately my enthusiasm and devotion to my work always outweighed my body hatred.

One Thanksgiving, on a trip home from Providence, I spotted the name Jack Wiener in *The New York Times*. My boyfriend from that magical summer in Connecticut two years earlier had made it. He was now dancing professionally in New York. I chanced a call. He remembered me . . . and we made a date for the following day. There I was, all bosom and buttocks, thirty-five pounds more of me than the last time we had been together. I was scared that he would be turned off by my size. Instead, he was turned on, big time.

We reconnected, this time not as a dance duo but as a couple. Jack proposed marriage that Christmas and we married the following June.

In the two months before the big event, I whittled my weight down to 130 pounds so I'd look ravishing in my silk wedding gown. I looked like a princess, even beautiful. Yet I was so dizzy that I fainted at the ceremony. Everyone thought it was the excitement. In truth, I had been starving myself for weeks . . . and the Merry Widow that nipped my waist into shape was cutting off my air supply.

After my marriage, I taught dance in the New York City public schools. I concealed my curvaceous hips with wraparound dance skirts over my leotards. Since I looked like most of the teachers I had studied with, clad in a leotard with a modest dance skirt tied at my waist—and my students loved me—I was able to hold my self-doubt in check. I was married; I was a successful teacher. I had proof that I was *okay*.

But no matter how successful I was as a teacher, a wife, a woman, I could never totally distract myself for any period of time from my discontent with my body image. It didn't matter that people would say,

"Hattie, you look great. What's your problem? If I had your body I'd be thrilled . . . and so would my husband!"

I started bingeing, eating whole pies at one sitting, whole jars of peanut butter with a spoon. My emotional hunger was insatiable. This time I tried vomiting to control my weight. It didn't work. I was unable to find relief in purging. And by dressing carefully, I somehow always managed to look thin.

I became pregnant with my son Joshua in the third year of my marriage. In a class for expectant mothers I met singer Elly Stone, a neighbor, who was expecting her son Matthew. From Elly, I learned about the hazards of preservatives and chemicals in foods and how whole grains and fresh, organically grown fruits and vegetables contribute to total health.

Pregnancy may have ballooned my body to a fully rounded 145 pounds, but knowing I was bearing a child shifted my concern from how I looked to my health, and the health of my child. All thought of binge eating and purging disappeared. Since 1963, when Joshua was born, I have been intent on eating properly. I even played a major role in the success of the Greenhouse, New York's first organic food co-op, and was instrumental in getting Chinese restaurants throughout New York City to offer brown rice—a healthier alternative to processed white rice.

While my health consciousness had been raised, I was still dissatisfied with the changes in my body. Whatever muscle tone and shape I had achieved by dancing had been supplanted by post-pregnancy stretch marks and post-nursing sagging breasts. Once again, I envisioned myself turning before my very eyes into one of the steam-room ladies.

Two years later, when my daughter Rama was born, I was better prepared for the shock. Resigning myself to how matronly I felt, I decided to concentrate on being healthy and to dress pretty, work hard, be a nice person and a terrific mom. My energy and sense of humor would see me through. I smiled from the neck up as I sagged from the neck down.

I thrived on motherhood.

By this time, my husband and I had opened our highly successful School for Creative Movement on New York City's Upper West Side, where we taught several hundred students every year. I was dancing every day, and sharing my love of dance and movement with bright-eyed preschoolers.

Even with the admiration and respect I received from students and parents alike, my self-image remained very negative. When I looked in the mirror, I still compared myself to dancers I saw on stage and models in magazines. I was sure that they had no physical imperfections, no flaws of the flesh. I felt like a loser. A roly-poly loser at that.

Once again I launched a quest for the perfect body, trying every diet, every exercise gimmick I could get my hands on. I used my bathroom scale like a Geiger counter to detect the presence of the first trace of additional weight. I was on a teeter-totter. Up ten pounds, down ten pounds. Fat wardrobe, thin wardrobe. There was no peace.

By the time my daughter turned sixteen, she was a gorgeous young woman with radiant skin and an athletic, naturally thin body, taut buttocks and strong, lithe limbs. I constantly compared my body to her dewy skin and slim hips. I became obsessed with jealousy for my own child and it made me thoroughly nauseated.

This painful realization that I was competing with my beloved daughter Rama was a powerful wake-up call. It propelled my decision to learn to cherish my body through its changes so that I would never again be plagued by envy and self-disgust. This wasn't just another New Year's resolution or a good idea that I might or might not follow. This decision touched the core of my being. By conquering these negative traits, I would develop the courage to master whatever challenges life delivered to me.

And if I was going to learn to cherish my body, I'd better develop a body worthy of this esteem. I knew I would never have the body of a teenager again, yet I was certain I could have the flexibility, stamina and joy of life I remembered from my youth.

I observed my own children and the little ones I taught. They were alive! They had no preconceptions or expectations about how anyone, including me, should look or behave. Unencumbered by preconceptions and doubts, they were happy with their bodies and simply did what felt good. If they wanted to jump, they jumped; if they felt like taking a nap, they did, and their bodies were healthy and fit. They were adorable.

Surely I had felt that way once. What had happened to make me so uncomfortable with my own body, to lose that sheer sense of joy at being alive? Here I was, a successful wife, mother and teacher who was continually told I was attractive, yet I felt like a sham.

I was only in my mid-thirties, yet I was consumed with fears of becoming fat, ugly and old. The psychic pain became unbearable. I decided to use therapy to reach back to the source of my feelings of self-loathing, determined to gain self-respect and to shed my obsession with weight and aging.

I may have begun my quest fixated on youth and beauty, but guided by my therapist, I grew away from this shallow, narcissistic way of being. It may sound corny but I stopped caring about the size of my thighs and started concentrating on the size of my heart. The more I loved and cared for others, the more respect I gained for myself.

And, miraculously, the more attractive I became.

This awakening inspired me to become a therapist so I could help others. I continued teaching and incorporated dance into my practice, becoming a dance therapist. It was hardly a surprise that the women—and even the men—who came to me for treatment wanted to eliminate the same negative body image issues that once plagued me. At last all that pain and agony I had been through could be put to good use!

In contrast to my professional success, my personal life was in turmoil. My son was in college and my daughter was on her way, when my husband of twenty-five years announced that he believed a divorce was the only solution to our problems. Undercurrents of discontent had been with us for years and our arguments had become more and more frequent, so I was not taken by complete surprise by his decision.

Still, it was painful. For me, divorce was an admission of failure, and the prospect of starting a whole new life on my own was terrifying. I wept and wailed, consumed with self-pity for about a year. You might say I had a relapse of narcissism. Then, quite candidly, it hit me that, of all the things in my marriage, the thing I missed most was our sexual intimacy. So I started dating.

I had been out of the dating loop for more than half of my life. Where to begin? Things had changed since my last fling as a single woman. I talked to friends and went to the places where suitable, eligible men might be. Maybe my ex-husband didn't think I was terrific anymore, but I was intent on proving that other men didn't share his opinion. I had a ball. I was so distracted by all this exciting male attention that my body obsessions faded into the background . . . at least for a while.

"Personals" had become popular, so I started reading—and answering—ads in *New York* magazine and *The Village Voice* that struck my fancy. I had some fabulous experiences out of this, receiving a few marriage proposals from older guys who didn't appeal to me and propositions from younger men who did.

Though I was intent on finding another husband, it wasn't happening. Like it or not, I was on my own. That's when I realized that simply having a man wasn't the answer. It would take much more work to become the woman I had to be for the rest of my life. Something inside of me still had to be healed. This started my spiritual quest.

I found before me a cornucopia of wonderful experiences and philosophies that I had never explored. I set out to try them all. I wasn't obsessed, I was *determined*. I tried everything: chiropractors, New Age healers, the Forum, shiatsu, yoga, rolfing, reinvention, aromatherapy, homeopathy, crystals, vitamin therapy, herbs, meditation and massages.

I zealously scanned newspapers and bulletin boards in search of answers. I took classes, workshops and seminars and even intense, one-on-one work with a spiritual coach who taught me about visualization and manifestation.

I assure you these were not the actions of a dilettante in search of adventure or a feel-good junkie out for a quick fix. As they say, when the pupil is ready, the teacher shows up. I was ready—and wonderful, loving teachers and healers came into my life to guide me.

Soon, I started looking, feeling and acting as I had when I was at the High School for Performing Arts, dancing the mambo in the lunchroom alongside Arthur Mitchell—future director of the Dance Theatre of Harlem—and Suzanne Pleshette, who was destined to become a famous actress. Friends and clients who witnessed my metamorphosis wondered what was happening. They were certain that I had had a facelift or discovered a doctor who was pumping me full of youth serum, or that I had tapped the Fountain of Youth. They assumed that I had to have done something drastic because I looked—and acted—younger and more alive than they had seen me in years. They demanded that I give them the name of my plastic surgeon and tell them what youth elixir I was taking. When I replied that I hadn't had surgery and the closest thing to an elixir I ever swallowed was fresh carrot juice, they were stunned.

Before long, I was sharing my secrets with a few friends. They too started growing younger. Now I had tangible proof. What I had done for myself was no accident. The changes I had made in my own diet, body-work and attitude were producing the same remarkable results in the people who were following in my footsteps.

Encouraged by these successes, I selectively introduced my newly proven anti-aging techniques into my therapy practice. A year later, psychotherapy took a back seat to my work with anti-aging. The seeds of RetroAging were germinating.

Then, one day in 1988, when I was fifty-two, I entered the Roseland Over-50 Bathing Suit Beauty Contest on a lark and won first prize. I never planned to be a beauty queen. I had gone to Roseland merely as an antidote to sadness. My daughter had embarked for China the night before and, alone and crying, I spotted a notice about the contest in the newspaper. I tucked my sexiest swimsuit into my bag—in case I decided to join in the competition.

Since dancing always makes me feel good, I figured I could shake the blues just by being there. Other people, when seeing me dance, encouraged me to enter. They said I was a sure winner.

I was as shocked at winning as I was at how people were inspired by me.

The morning after, I brazenly walked onto the *Regis & Kathie Lee* set wearing the same skimpy swimsuit I'd worn in the contest. Regis, pretending to faint, declared, "Omigod! Hattie! There she is—an inspiration to all America."

And the *New York Daily News* ran a huge photo of me with the headline "Golden Boldie" and raved, "Wiener makes Cher look like John Candy on a bad day."

My son, who had just returned from vacationing in Mexico, called and said, "Ma, tell me it's not true. My friend called to tell me that my own mother appeared almost naked on national television." Guess what picture got tacked to the bulletin board over his desk?

This public recognition broke through my reluctance to tell everyone what I was doing to keep my own body in shape. I do such zany things—like hammering away my cellulite with a rubber mallet—that I was afraid people would think I was a kook. Far from it. Every time I told someone about this, they raced to the hardware store so they could thump for themselves!

Two years after winning at Roseland, my daughter Rama and I both appeared in bikinis on *The Sally Jessy Raphael Show* about mothers who look as great in swimsuits as their grown daughters: she, magnificently fit and trim; me, thirty years her senior, shapely, strong and sexy. The audience applauded appreciatively when we hugged and kissed on the set. What a wonderful feeling it was for us to openly share our mutual warmth and respect—especially on national TV.

And two years after that, beyond even *my* wildest dreams, I was first runner-up in a bikini contest in the Caribbean, beating out twenty-year-olds!

Youth isn't the same for everyone. You have to decide what being young is for you. It may be as simple as changing the color of your hair or learning how to skate. For me, it meant relocating to the Caribbean island of Tortola, learning to scuba dive and dancing reggae all night.

In my two magical years in paradise, I became more in touch with my healing powers and even more determined to share with the world what I had discovered about reversing aging. I returned to New York, where I expanded my anti-aging practice, achieving remarkable results with my clients, both women and men.

When the men started to see the women in their lives getting younger, they broke down and admitted that they were afraid of aging too. As one said, "Old age may be a state of mind, but what I saw in the mirror was driving me crazy. I thought it would never happen, but I was turning into my dad before my very eyes. Thanks, Hattie; I'm me again!"

Now, as I enter my sixties, I respect myself totally. I am fascinated with the aging process and no longer fear the effects of time. RetroAge grew out of my journey from self-loathing to self-love, a love that eventually transcends self.

2 THE BIG BLITZ

GETTING OFF TO A CLEAN START

The first step to growing younger is clearing away the past. This means getting rid of everything that does not positively impact your health and well-being.

Even the neatest, most organized person has a store of items—clothing, shoes, cosmetics, books, even foods—that have been put aside in an "I'll-need-this-someday" fashion. I say these possessions keep us stuck to the past and hold us back from a youth-filled future.

Wouldn't you want to hide in embarrassment if your mother, or your best friend, knew what you had stowed away in those storage boxes under your bed, or about the gallon of chocolate–chocolate chip ice cream wrapped in foil and stashed behind the frozen peas?

And what about those shoe boxes on the top shelf in your bedroom closet? The ones with the cookies and chocolates nestled in tissue paper so no one will see the contents should they pop the lids. Or the steamer trunk filled with clothes you're certain you'll be able to wear again. Or the boxes of pictures of the one who broke your heart . . . twenty years ago.

Every one of us has hideaways where we stash our secrets. Some hide the special binge foods that we eat only behind closed doors, with the curtains drawn and nobody else around. Others hide clothes, letters, photographs—all those things we know we no longer need but somehow resist getting rid of. Someday we'll get around to it.

With the Blitz, someday is *now*.

Don't panic. I know how hard it is to tackle those piles of papers and magazines you've been meaning to read. And why *should* you get rid of those fabulous "skinny" clothes? They once made you feel like a million bucks. Besides, you'll lose that weight and be wearing them again one of these days. Right?

Yeah, right.

One of these days. Like *someday,* that's a catchphrase that holds us back. Hanging on to the past—materially or emotionally—does not make us young; it keeps us stuck in the past.

Frankly, this is common sense. How can we move forward if we're clutching the remnants of days gone by? Blitzing is a powerful, proactive technique that frees us from age-making foods, possessions and, ultimately, habits. It sets the stage for RetroAging.

A Blitz is the dynamite that will blast you out of the past. Once freed of residual clutter, you are ready to create a youth-filled future.

EXACTLY WHAT IS A BLITZ?

A Blitz is a systematic clean-up of *every* aspect of your environment. With RetroAging, you will blitz every area of your life that you have cluttered with past "I can't do withouts." But don't worry, you don't have to do it all at once, right now. You can Blitz in stages as we go through the four steps of RetroAging. I suggest that you tackle your kitchen while you are working on Step 1—Eating; your wardrobe, in tandem with Step 2—Exercise; the bathroom, with Step 3—Skincare, and everything else as you work on Step 4—Attitude.

Believe it or not, Blitzes are fun, once you get over your initial fear that you may be opening Fibber Magee's closet—or Pandora's box.

Yes, there will be things that are difficult, even painful, to face, but once you get into the process you will experience great freedom and lightness. After all, possessions are merely *things*. It's not as if that dress or tuxedo you wore to your senior prom *is* that prom. The prom was then; this is now. You have the memories in your heart, where they should be. You don't need that mass of tulle and taffeta or that too-tight brocade jacket and ruffled shirt to remind you of your youth.

When we hold on to the possessions of our past, youth becomes a memory, not a possibility. That's exactly what we want to avoid. RetroAging puts youth in the future, where it belongs. Blitzes clear the way.

PHASE 1: GETTING READY

When you begin a Blitz, you have to set the stage:

- Set aside a block of time—at least three hours—for each Blitz. You may need two trips down Memory Lane before you can part with the contents of your cupboards and closets.
- Put on the most comfortable clothes you own. Nothing fancy, mind you—a Blitz is definitely down and dirty.
- Turn on your favorite radio station or pop in that special tape. Upbeat is best; Gregorian chants tend to slow you down!
- Break out a new box of super-strength jumbo garbage bags and any other supplies you think you may need to clean up in your wake. You may want to have a box of tissues handy to dry your tears. Getting rid of the past can be traumatic.

You may find it helpful to enroll a friend or two to partner with you in this project. Just make sure they are people who have a sense of humor and will hold you to the spirit of the Blitz. You don't want someone who'll let you rationalize saving 75 percent of the stuff you have just mustered the courage to part with.

If you're intimidated by the prospect of letting even your closest friends see what you have behind those closed doors, you can go it alone. You may find it helpful to "bookend" your work by calling a friend on the phone before and after your cleanup. You'll have the benefits of a friend's support without actually showing what you've been hiding.

Personally, I find it more productive, not to mention a lot more fun, to have company. I still remember my sympathetic friends who listened without judgment as I tearfully showed them my prized possessions, treasures from my past, and explained why I couldn't live without a certain book, a "Marilyn Monroe dress," the gallons of Breyer's toasted almond and chocolate ice cream in my freezer. Pretty soon, we all were doubling over with laughter as we filled bag after bag with *stuff*. They helped me to break free of my past and I am forever grateful to them.

PHASE 2: THE BLITZ PROCESS

This may be the hardest part of RetroAging. We know we must change how we eat and start a specific program of exercise if we are to turn back the clock, but rearranging the kitchen cabinets and working on our wardrobes . . . well, that's another matter altogether. That's *personal*.

Resist the temptation to slam the door on your clutter and reach for a chocolate bar. Just because you bought something doesn't mean you have to eat it, wear it or save it for a rainy day. Get into the habit of getting rid of stuff that doesn't serve you. After all, where would you rather see that cherry-cheese danish: in the garbage or on your hips? Think of Blitzing as merely another aspect of recycling.

If it is too appalling to throw into the trash an outfit that doesn't fit and doesn't become you, donate it to charity, give it to a neighbor, sell it on consignment—get it out of your space!

In all probability, you will not be able to make a complete Blitz in one fell swoop. Most of us can't. The shock of going from a cupboard laden with pasta and cookies and a fridge filled with cans of cola and condiment bottles to a kitchen filled with brown rice, whole grain breads and fresh vegetables can traumatize even the staunchest youth-seeker. But believe it or not, it can be done. Just follow this system and soon Blitzing will be as natural as brushing your teeth.

The process of elimination is simple. Sort items—be they kitchen staples or clothing—into three categories:

Automatic Throwaways   Things you don't have to think twice about keeping. Do this quickly or you may talk yourself into hanging on to them even longer.

Possible Keepers   Items that would haunt you if you merely threw them away, though in your heart you suspect you really should part with them. With these, ask yourself if you have used these items in the past six months and if you really will be needing them in the six months ahead. If the answer is no in either direction, get rid of them.

Definite Keepers   These are the items that you truly cherish; foods that nourish both body and soul; clothing that makes you look and feel sensational; possessions that reflect a sense of self-worth. This process does not happen overnight, but if you dedicate yourself to RetroAging, this will soon be the only category left.

Be patient with yourself. After all, streamlining or downsizing may not be new concepts in the corporate world, but we do not naturally apply them to our personal lives.

I must confess that it took years for me to reach the point where I am today. After my divorce, I was forced to face twenty-five years of memories and material possessions. While it was frightening at the time, I am grateful that this set me on a new course. Now the same friends who watched me agonize over getting rid of the trappings of my past call me the Blitz Queen. Some even threaten to nail their cupboards and closets shut before I visit.

Today my life is rich, even though my possessions are, by any standard, few. My eating and fitness habits are enviable. My energy is boundless. Thanks to Blitzing, I am free to move into a future unfettered by clutter.

PHASE 3: STARTING OVER

After you have taken the first cut at the clutter in your life, such as the kitchen, you must be conscious of a few pitfalls. Blitzing is not yet a habit, therefore you may find yourself facing a lot of space begging to be filled.

Don't go rushing off to the nearest supermarket to replenish your food supply. You will not starve. I promise you. Pretty soon, your cupboards will be full again, only now the macaroni and cheese and potato chips will be replaced by foods that will nourish your body, not destroy it. The next chapter will teach you how to eat for youth.

As for everything else, get ready to Blitz a clear path for an exciting future.

Move from your kitchen to your wardrobe, keeping in mind that everything in your closet was purchased by the person you once were, not the one you're aspiring to be. As you shed your former self-image, you will become ready to create a whole new, younger you—complete with an attractive, updated wardrobe.

I'm not saying to throw *everything* but the hangers away. In all probability, that would not be economically sound. I am, however, assuring you that clearing the boards allows you to dress in a fresh, youthful fashion. For example, you may still need to wear corporate garb to the office, but you don't have to limit yourself to drab colors and stuffy styles. You men may change the colors of your shirts or add an unexpectedly wild tie. Women may shorten their skirts and show more leg than they ever dared.

One of my earliest clients emerged from her Blitzes like a butterfly from a chrysalis. This fifty-five-year-old nurse-midwife, who wore hospital scrubs at work, traded in her rather sedate, even dowdy, personal wardrobe for a series of sensational ensembles befitting her youthful, spirited persona.

Even if you wind up keeping many of the clothes in your closet, you will see them differently after the Blitz, combining and accessorizing them in brand-new ways.

When I first restyled my look, I tried an experiment: I asked the twenty-year-old salesclerk at a trendy SoHo shop to choose a dress and accessories for me. She brought out a *very* sexy backless white cotton outfit made in Italy and dangling rhinestone earrings. I was sure that this look was wrong for me, especially at my age, but I reminded myself that this was only a game. I didn't have to buy it; I just had to try it. I did. When I parted the dressing room curtains and walked into the store, I actually inspired oos and ahs from other customers. A month later, I wore this same ensemble on national TV after winning the Roseland Over-50 Bathing Beauty Contest. I still get compliments on those earrings. As for the white outfit . . . it's been replaced by a slinky black minidress with tiny spaghetti straps.

Before long, Blitzing will have become second nature, something you do any time you find yourself bogged down or overwhelmed. So go for it. It works like a charm to lift your spirits and move you forward.

Together we will Blitz through your kitchen, your wardrobe, your bathroom, your work space—anywhere you have stashed stuff. You'll find Blitz charts at the end of each of the chapters dealing with the Four Steps of RetroAging. I suggest photocopying these blank forms and keeping a notebook to chronicle your progress. Once you cultivate this habit, you'll find yourself Blitzing over and over again.

3 STEP 1: EATING

NOURISH YOUR WAY TO YOUTH

Get ready for an unexpected adventure. Now you're going to take Step 1 and learn how to eat! I know, you've been feeding yourself for years, but how much of what you've consumed was really benefiting your body? The nutritional program you're about to learn divides what you eat into two categories: (1) Foods, which contribute to your youthfulness—not to mention your health and vitality—and (2) Non-Foods, which are of little nutritional value or just downright destructive. With RetroAge Eating, you will also master the art of food combining, a style of eating for your whole life that assures efficient digestion and maximum nutrition, and is completely satisfying. What could be better?

Perhaps you thought that the English muffin topped with sugar-free jam and low-fat margarine you had with your water-processed decaffeinated coffee with skim milk and artificial sweetener this morning was healthy eating. While you certainly had plenty to eat, according to this program, there wasn't a single nourishing food on your plate. In fact, this meal leaves your body starving for nutrition and flooded with toxins.

If you happen to be that one person in the world who eats only fruits, vegetables and whole grains, never craves desserts or pizza, and thinks chocolate bars are bricks, you can skip this step and jump ahead to Step 2—Exercise, with my compliments . . . and envy.

But if you're like almost everyone else on this planet, myself included, you'll have to master new techniques to keep ahead of aging. After two decades of testing an awesome array of diets and eating styles, I've come up with a nutritional program that will make the difference between whether you are thin or heavy, strong or weak, vital or debilitated, young or old.

I suspect what usually steers us away from healthy eating is our fear that we'll be sentenced to munching oat bran and alfalfa sprouts for the rest of our lives. Nothing could be further from the truth. You'll be eating *mounds* of delicious, satisfying foods without feeling the least bit deprived.

In the course of reversing my own aging, I radically altered my food intake. That meant systematically identifying and eliminating whatever foods caused me to be sluggish, bloated and chronically tired. I also realized the more I ate of these foods, the more ravenous I became. I'm not just talking about wanting to eat again an hour after a Chinese dinner either. My appetite was taking over my life. As much as I ate, I never seemed to be satisfied. I was filling my stomach with sweets and other "comfort foods" that I loved without meeting my body's nutritional needs.

Sound familiar?

To get to the root of this feeding frenzy, I began to experiment. I started by keeping track of what, when and why I ate. Pretty soon, I was able to see patterns emerging. Candy made me crave salty foods, like popcorn or chips; coffee made me crave muffins; meat made me crave desserts. It was as though, in some peculiar way, my body was attempting to balance itself out but was making strangely unhealthy choices.

While these tasty treats may have given me instant gratification, within no time I felt as though a monster had taken possession of my body. I ate more and more of my favorite foods in hopes of satisfying my insatiable hunger. My brain was telling me to stop, but I kept reaching for things that were detrimental to my body and my life. There I was, stuck in a dilemma! I needed food to survive, yet almost everything I ate set off a feeding frenzy.

This started me on a search for a whole new way of eating. I didn't know it at the time, but the principles of RetroAge Eating were germinating.

ABOUT EATING

1. Don't weigh yourself more than once every few days; resist the tendency to get on a scale. It's how you feel and look that's important, not the numbers.
2. Don't think of this as a diet. Think of it as a new way of eating for the rest of your life.
3. Never skip meals to make up for overeating or to lose weight or inches quickly.
   Drastically cutting food intake slows down metabolism and makes you ravenously hungry.
4. Don't be ashamed to admit to yourself (and others) what you're actually eating. Feeling guilty won't help you lose weight and develop good eating habits. It's self-respect that keeps you thin and healthy.
5. Be prepared to be overly involved with food and eating—your entire relationship to food will be questioned as you adopt this new health-giving style of eating.
6. Locate restaurants that serve delicious, healthy food. This will make it easier for you to get the foods your body wants and needs when dining out.
7. Eat foods as close to their pure, unprocessed, unrefined form as possible for maximum nutritive benefit. Buy as many organically grown foods as your budget allows. Not only is this great for your body, it also creates a demand and supports chemical-free, naturally composted farming, which is good for our environment!
8. Whenever you eliminate a Non-Food, replace it with something healthy and tasty that you love.
9. Eat until you're satisfied. If you don't, you risk triggering a binge.
10. Remember the Hattietude:
    Deprivation Backfires,
    Satisfaction Inspires.

By process of elimination, I found that, while some foods—like hamburgers, chicken and rice, pepperoni pizza, desserts—made me feel bloated and out of sorts, other foods—curried vegetables on brown and wild rice pilaf, whole-grain pasta with a simple garlic and basil-filled tomato sauce (no cheese or meat), luscious mixed vegetable salads and fruits—revved me up with boundless energy. Once I noticed a pattern emerging, I kept track of which foods fueled my body and which slowed me down.

I needed a specific plan of attack to keep me on target or I would inadvertently slip back into sloppy eating. My strategy was to label everything that triggered my binges and mood swings *Non-Foods* and reserve the term *Food* only for those things that truly nourished my body. When I say *Non-Foods*, I'm not referring to the shelves and shelves of inedible things like paper towels and floor wax that your grocer's cash register calls Non-Foods. I'm referring to specific food products that deprive our bodies of health: sugared cereals; hot dogs and other processed meats; artificial sweeteners; artificial anything; white bread; cookies; candies; cakes; canned veggies; fruit-filled yogurt; frozen and canned juices . . . even white rice and pasta. *Foods* are fresh and whole, as close to their natural state as possible. This means whole grains rather than processed; fresh fruits and vegetables in season. I vowed to systematically eliminate all *Non-Foods* from my diet, no matter how difficult it was or how long it took.

This simple distinction has really worked for me and for my clients. It has served as a constant reminder to consciously weed out all those destructive "goodies" from our diets. As for me, I may never be able to *totally* eliminate them—at least I haven't so far—but Non-Foods now make up a considerably smaller part of my daily food consumption.

Why is it so difficult to stick to a healthy diet? This question keeps coming up with my clients as they work to clean up their eating. I explain to them that what we eat controls what we eat. While this may be an odd answer, it accurately describes this tailspinlike phenomenon:

- You start the day with the best of intentions: You won't eat sugary desserts or stuff yourself. You'll have only healthy foods in moderate quantity. In your mind, this seems entirely possible.
- Then what happens? You eat. And if even one of the foods on your plate is a Non-Food, the delicate chemical balance of your body is upset and your resolve flies right out the window.
- You're caught. The power of these Non-Foods is awesome. The what, when and why of your eating them will control the rest of your day, leaving you feeling sluggish, often aching and

tired, not to mention emotionally low. To make yourself feel better, you . . . eat. And I have yet to meet the person who turns to carrot sticks for comfort. The ice cream, the chocolate, the bag of chips just make us feel worse. And the cycle continues.

It's happened to all of us more times than we care to remember.

Binge eating may be rooted in emotional upset or stress, but the trigger is almost always food-related. The biochemical reaction caused by what we eat is that potent.

RetroAge Eating changes all that. With it, you will always have a powerful weapon to balance your cravings. Then, as soon as you realize you have gone into a tailspin, you will be able to identify what Non-Foods threw you off and get back to safe ground.

MIXING AND MATCHING THE FOODS YOU EAT

A primary component of RetroAge Eating is *Food Combining*. You may have heard this phrase before. Although it was popularized in the early eighties by Marilyn and Harvey Diamond's excellent best-seller *Fit for Life*, this concept was pioneered in the 1930s by William Howard Hay, M.D.

As I studied how my own body reacted to what I ate, I discovered that the only way I could eat to satisfaction and stay healthy and thin was to Food Combine. That meant never eating animal proteins—meat, cheese, eggs, yogurt, etc.—and starchy carbohydrates at the same meal. As long as I stuck to this regime, my weight stayed down and my energy stayed up. Any time I strayed, I started to feel and look awful. It became quite clear to me that as long as I put my health first, beauty followed. My skin looked radiant and alive, my eyes bright, and my hair shining. And I had boundless energy.

The effect of Food Combining was so powerful and positive for me that I made it an integral part of the bodywork program I was doing with my clients. Prior to this, I was simply emphasizing the nutritive value of food and helping them to eliminate empty calories and destructive fats from their diets.

I taught this system to my clients with great results, yet I never clearly understood the biochemistry behind the process. My lack of understanding bothered me. Then one day while discussing RetroAge Eating with a client who took great pleasure in resisting this part of his RetroAging program, he remarked, "This sounds a lot like how my mother cooked for me when I was a kid. In fact, I still have her favorite cookbook. I'll bring it to you."

Voilà! In two short pages, Dr. Hay made every aspect of Food Combining totally clear to me. The book, *The Official Cook Book of the Hay System*, by Esther L. Smith, with an introduction by William Howard Hay, M.D., is long out of print, first published by Pocono Haven, Mount Pocono, PA, in August 1934.

I was astounded and delighted. More than fifty years before I instructed my first client to make a list of the Foods and Non-Foods she ate, Dr. Hay wrote, in his introduction to the eleventh printing (October 1940):

A very large part of the foods ordinarily eaten are not food in any sense of the word, as food is replenishment material for the body. . . . Any so-called food that does not furnish what the body requires and can use is not to be considered as food at all, and many of these are positively harmful to the body. There are so many foods that do represent body needs that it is not necessary to introduce anything but these, yet not detract in the slightest degree from the perfection of any meal, from either the utility or the aesthetic pleasures of the table.

He summed up my Foods/Non-Foods concept in three sentences. What better corroboration could I find?

As to his theories of Food Combining, Dr. Hay wrote:

Foods are of vastly different sorts, also, as regards to the digestive requirements, some being digested largely in one part of the digestive tract while others digest in a different part, and the body modifies the digestive juices to suit the tasks at hand at the time.

Basically, foods are carbohydrates or proteins, each with vastly different digestive requirements, so different that they are even digested in separate parts of the system. Carbohydrates—cereals, potatoes, corn, pumpkins and dry fruits like dates and raisins—start digesting in the mouth, where ptyalin in the saliva splits them into dextroses (sugars), and then pass through the acidic stomach to continue the process in the alkaline medium found in the intestines. Proteins—meats, seafoods, cheese—need the strong gastric juices—pepsin and hydrochloric acid—found in the stomach to release their nutrients.

If carbohydrates and proteins are in the stomach at the same time, the stomach acids start the fermentation process on the carbohydrates, which interferes with protein digestion. The result is, according to Esther Smith, "chaos . . . fermentation, gas, acidosis . . . illness in one form or other."

No wonder we all feel so stuffed and out of sorts after Thanksgiving dinner!

To help my clients master the principles of Food Combining, I stripped it down to its simplest form. I called the Starchy Complex Carbohydrates and Vegetable Proteins Group 1 and Animal Proteins Group 2.

My sole instruction:

NEVER EAT FOODS FROM GROUP 1 WITH FOODS FROM GROUP 2.

Group 1—Starchy Complex Carbs and Vegetable Proteins Rice, wheat barley and other grains, beans and peas, potatoes, winter squashes, corn, bread, pasta, tofu, tempeh, chips, pretzels, cereals, raw nuts, seeds and nut butters.

When you eat starchy complex carbs, you can eat only vegetables, cooked or raw, including salad. Remember: Absolutely no animal protein, not even a splash of grated cheese, sour cream or yogurt.

Group 2—Animal Proteins Chicken, turkey, all fowl, fish (canned and fresh), beef, pork, veal, eggs, milk, cheese, yogurt and all milk products.

When you eat proteins, you can only eat non-starchy vegetables (anything not listed above) with them. Remember: Never have any starchy complex carbohydrate foods with your animal proteins.

You'll notice that these Food Combining concepts go against almost everything you learned about eating in school. And, for some incomprehensible reason, every single cuisine violates these principles. For example: chicken and rice, spaghetti and meatballs, chili con carne, pizza, franks and beans, steamed dumplings, Irish stew, sushi, burgers and fries . . . and, alas, just about every conceivable sandwich.

Two additional considerations: Never drink beverages, including water, with any of the above foods. Drinking with meals interferes with efficient digestion by diluting the stomach acids. Have your beverage a half hour before eating and wait an hour after.

Follow the same time table when eating fruit. You may have it a half hour before meals or one hour after meals. Fruit is digested so quickly that, if eaten with other foods, it starts fermentation in your system. It's no surprise that you'll get bloated and gassy . . . not to mention experiencing mood swings from the resulting elevated blood sugar.

THE INSIDE SKINNY ON FATS

Please note that I do not advocate a no-fat or radically low-fat diet. The body needs some fat to function properly. However, it's vital to substantially reduce animal fats. These fats—including dairy products—are hazardous, having been implicated as causes of cancer, heart attacks, you name it. One more reason for choosing a vegetarian diet is that all plant oils contain 0% cholesterol. Natural fats from nuts, avocados and vegetables, are safe in moderation. Stay away from, or avoid adding, fats of any kind—even vegetable fats—to your foods. And, of course, never ever ever eat fried foods, especially breaded fried foods.

Current Federal guidelines recommend that no more than 30 percent of our daily calories should be from fat, with no more than 10 percent in saturated fats. Many experts contend that the type of fat one consumes is as important as how much, and I agree.

Safest is monounsaturated fat, which comes from olive oil, avocados and nuts—especially almonds and hazelnuts. They help to lower dangerous LDL cholesterol and contain antioxidants that deter artery clogging and even chronic diseases such as cancer. Studies have shown that people whose main source of fat is olive oil live longer and have less heart disease and cancer (especially breast cancer) than those who consume other fats. Heating, however, may destroy some antioxidant activity in olive oil. Personally, I only use cold-pressed extra virgin olive oil for cooking and roasted sesame or extra virgin olive oil for all my salads, veggies and air-popped popcorn . . . my favorite late night treat. I use them in place of butter on cooked vegetables and sometimes on toast. They help my skin stay beautiful, and the pungent flavor is deliciously satisfying.

Also in this "healthy fat" category are the omega-3 fatty acids found in fish, especially salmon, herring, mackerel, sardines and tuna, and some plants and plant oils, including canola, grapeseed and flaxseed oils, walnuts and walnut oil. I recommend a daily intake of one teaspoon of flaxseed oil to enhance the immune system.

Canola oil, which is especially low in saturated fat, high in monounsaturated fat and amazingly rich in youth-giving omega-3 fatty acids, is extremely versatile as it can be used not just in salad dressings but also for sautéing or stir-frying or in any recipe that calls for cooking oil. Rare, but terrific, macadamia nut oil, found in health food stores, is the highest in monounsaturated fat of all salad oils.

Polyunsaturated fats, found in soybean and corn oil, margarine, shortening and mayonnaise, may help lower cholesterol; however, they are also prone to cause detrimental free-radical chemical reactions, which cause aging, so should be avoided. Another minus: Many polyunsaturated fats are hydrogenated, or hardened, which means they are high in trans-fatty acids, which contribute to heart disease and increased cholesterol levels.

We have long known that saturated fats, which come from animal products—meats, poultry skin, cream and whole milk, butter, cheeses and full-fat yogurt—promote heart disease by boosting cholesterol and clogging arteries. They are also associated with an increase in certain cancers, most notably prostate and colon.

Add corn, safflower and sunflower seed oils as well as palm and coconut oils—tropical fats—to your list of dangerous fats. While corn,
safflower and sunflower seed oils have beneficial qualities, they are
high in dangerous omega-6 fatty acids, which can promote cancer, in-
flammatory reactions and immune system malfunctions. Unlike other
vegetable fats, which have little or no saturated fats, coconut and palm
oils are between 50 and 85 percent saturated fat. The body has diffi-
culty assimilating these, which accelerates aging.

As if you need one more reason to keep your fat intake low, one
gram of fat is nine calories while one gram of protein or carbohydrate
has only four calories. While we're on that topic, keep your protein intake low as well. Contrary to popular belief, excess protein can make
you fat, and it puts strain on your already overworked liver. Stick with
whole grains, vegetables and fruits. They'll keep you svelte and energetic.

STARTING YOUR RETRoAGE EATING PROGRAM

Now that you've been introduced to the concepts of Foods/Non-Foods
and Food Combining, you're ready to start reversing your aging process
with the RetroAge Eating program.

> **DON'T WORRY, YOU WON'T HAVE TO MAKE
> DRASTIC CHANGES
> IN THE WAY YOU EAT ALL AT ONCE.**
> *RetroAge Eating happens in stages.*

You begin by keeping an eating diary. As you write down everything you consume each day, you will graphically identify the Foods
and Non-Foods you eat on a regular basis. Even so-called "real" foods,
like that English muffin I mentioned earlier, can throw your body off
balance because it's made with white flour and refined sugar. By the
time you complete this chapter, you'll be pinpointing all health-giving
Foods on your plate as well as Non-Foods that can trigger a tailspin.

RETROAGE EATING BASICS

These instructions form the foundation of RetroAge Eating. The more you follow them, the younger you will look and feel! After all, that is the purpose of RetroAging, isn't it?

- **Master** the Principles of Food Combining.
  When Food Combining becomes second nature, you won't have to keep thinking about what you're going to eat to grow young, you'll reach for the appropriate foods naturally.
- **Identify** all Foods and Non-Foods in your current diet. Once you make the distinction between Foods, which build health and reverse aging, and Non-Foods, which steal youth and vitality, you can begin to eliminate what's aging you from your diet.
- **Enrich** your diet with *raw* vegetables, salads and fruit. Including raw veggies and salads at *every* meal provides your body with the powerful enzymes it needs for effective digestion. Fresh whole fruit and juices between meals round out the process. Remember, do not have fruit or juices in combination with any other food. You may have them a half an hour before meals and one hour after meals.
- **Avoid** drinking any liquid—even water—with meals.
  Fluids dilute the strong acid medium of the stomach and hamper the extraction of nutrients from your food. Wait a half hour after drinking to eat; an hour after eating to drink.
- **Detoxify** by drinking eight large glasses of filtered or spring water, herb or green tea daily. Your liver, kidneys and bladder need cleansing. An ample fluid supply makes that possible.

You'll experience improved digestion. Your metabolism will increase and your energy level will soar. Imagine that!

It feels wonderful to gain control over your intake of Non-Foods that steal your youth. If you don't, you will spend your life losing and gaining weight, experimenting with one diet after another and feeling like a failure. I know what I'm talking about. I've tried virtually every diet and weight-loss gimmick ever invented. With one, I ate so much pineapple I felt like a piña colada.

I may have lost weight initially with each of these routines, but the pounds always came back and I was left angry, frustrated and full of self-loathing.

One of my early clients, a New York–based TV-video producer in his late forties, was preoccupied with food, compulsively stuffing his body with unhealthy foods. He always had a can of soda or cup of coffee with cream and sugar in his hand and a drawer filled with gooey snacks within easy reach.

Since working with me, he has tossed out all the sodas and junk foods that once filled his kitchen, replacing them with yogurt, stone-ground wheat crackers, fresh vegetables and fruit. He still has a large appetite, but now he confines it to the healthy foods he combines for a well-balanced diet. He no longer dreads the effects of aging as he feels himself becoming more energetic and more optimistic. He is armed with the ability to take the actions to continuously claim his life. More importantly, he has started to love himself.

"When Hattie had me clean out my cupboards and closets and throw away everything she called Non-foods, I wanted to tie her up and gag her. How could I live without my chocolate cake and Diet Cokes?" he recalls. "Her inspiration and humor have enabled me to finally have the motivation to stick to my diet. I may not be as slim and trim as I dreamed of being, but I feel strong and healthy and have energy to spare. RetroAge has given me a whole new way of eating and I'm thrilled about that. I believe in my power to take charge of my life now."

KEEPING A FOOD DIARY

Before you can change the way you eat, you'll need to be aware *of what you are already eating.* That's where your Daily Eating Diary comes into play. Starting today, you will keep a log of *everything* you eat and drink for the next seven days. This is not an ordinary food journal. It is designed specifically to make you conscious of your relationship with the food you eat, not just the food itself.

You may want to photocopy these diary pages to carry with you during the day so you won't have to rely on your memory—and, admit it, to keep you honest. We tend to forget those lethal little snacks we indulge in when we need a boost.

Here's how it works: As soon as you eat anything—a meal, a snack or those cups of coffee at work—*immediately* note the day, date and time; what and how much you ate; and the *reason* for eating. This last item is an important part of the diary because it makes you aware of *why* you're eating what you're eating. The time of day may be 7 A.M. and the reason for eating is that it's breakfast time, but then again, it could be 2 A.M. and you're eating because you had an argument with your spouse right before you went to bed and you're still wrestling with your frustration . . . or it's 9 P.M. and you're sitting in front of the TV mindlessly munching after a frustrating day.

One important warning: Record *everything* that goes into your mouth. That includes what you taste while cooking dinner "just to make sure the seasoning's right" and that frozen yogurt or candy bar you had as a pick-me-up while you were racing to the bank. You may discover, as one surprised client did, that she had not been listing anything she ate standing up—such as a slice of pizza at the pizza parlor counter or the leftovers from the fridge. In fact, most of the time, she was barely aware that she had eaten these things. For her, if she wasn't sitting at a table and eating off a plate, it didn't count. She was startled at the quantity of calories she consumed in this unconscious state.

"When I started working with Hattie, I was absolutely convinced that my metabolism had been shut down by years of fad diets and diet pills," she notes. "Yes, I had slowed my body down by these unhealthy practices, but that wasn't the biggest cause of my weight gain. It took keeping this food diary and then learning Hattie's RetroAge Eating program to get my body into balance so that I could not only lose weight but get healthy as well."

Resist the temptation to edit your diary. You're the only one who'll see it. Don't make yourself "wrong" or indulge in guilt because you ate an entire pint of ice cream in one sitting. Everyone overeats from time to time, even disciplined dancers and athletes. If you ate it or drank it, write it down. Tell the truth, even if it's embarrassing. I assure you, it'll help you in the long run.

At the end of each day, read over your diary to identify your eating patterns. On Day 4, go back to Day 1 and circle all the Foods you ate and mark all the Non-Foods with Xes. From then on, you will do this every day, tallying your circles and crosses, to track your progress.

DAILY EATING DIARY
(SAMPLE)

What Eaten—Amount	Day Time	Reason for Eating (Notes on activities, emotions, circumstances)
8 oz. O J (frozen) Toasted sesame bagel with scallion cream cheese 2 mugs coffee, cream and sweetener	Monday Breakfast time 8:45 a.m.	Picked up at corner deli Ate at desk Opened mail as ate
Almond Danish Coffee, cream and sweetener	10:30 a.m.	"Coffee break" I guess I ate because it was there
Tuna salad with iceberg lettuce and mayonnaise on kaiser roll Large Diet Pepsi	2 p.m.	Lunch hour
Large Diet Pepsi	4 p.m.	Pick-me-upper . . . I need energy to make it through this afternoon. This job is so tedious.
2 8-ounce margaritas Bowl of taco chips; small bowl of salsa	5:45 p.m.	Met Mary for drinks after work. There are so many great-looking guys here. I'm nervous.
Large bowl vegetarian chili Mixed green salad— oil and vinegar 2 pint mugs of Sangria 1 cup Cappuccino with cocoa and sugar	8 p.m.	Dinner time . . . ate at Mexican restaurant with Mary. I'm glad her music career is taking off. I'm very tired.
1 bag butter-flavored microwave popcorn	12:30 a.m.	There's a good movie on TV. I wanted a bedtime snack.

DAILY TALLY:

FOODS: ___6___   NON-FOODS: ___17___

When your circles dominate your page, you'll know that you're well on your way to RetroAge Eating for age reversal. You'll understand why there are so few Foods on this sample chart once you learn the Principles of Food Combining.

DAILY EATING DIARY

DAY 1

DATE: _____

What Eaten—Amount	Day Date Time	Reason for Eating (Notes on activities, emotions, circumstances)

DAILY TALLY:

FOODS: _____   NON-FOODS: _____

DAILY EATING DIARY

DAY 2

DATE: _____

What Eaten—Amount	Day Date Time	Reason for Eating (Notes on activities, emotions, circumstances)

DAILY TALLY:

Foods: _____   Non-Foods: _____

DAILY EATING DIARY

DAY 3

DATE: _____

What Eaten—Amount	Day Date Time	Reason for Eating (Notes on activities, emotions, circumstances)

DAILY TALLY:

FOODS: _____   NON-FOODS: _____

DAILY EATING DIARY

DAY 4

DATE: _____

What Eaten—Amount	Day Date Time	Reason for Eating (Notes on activities, emotions, circumstances)

DAILY TALLY:

FOODS: _____   NON-FOODS: _____

DAILY EATING DIARY

DAY 5

DATE: _____

What Eaten—Amount	Day Date Time	Reason for Eating (Notes on activities, emotions, circumstances)

DAILY TALLY:

FOODS: _____   NON-FOODS: _____

DAILY EATING DIARY

DAY 6

DATE: _____

What Eaten—Amount	Day Date Time	Reason for Eating (Notes on activities, emotions, circumstances)

DAILY TALLY:

FOODS: _____   NON-FOODS: _____

DAILY EATING DIARY

DAY 7

DATE: _____

What Eaten—Amount	Day Date Time	Reason for Eating (Notes on activities, emotions, circumstances)

DAILY TALLY:

FOODS: _____   NON-FOODS: _____

RetroAge Eating has taken me more than twenty years to develop, and I still work at it daily. However, if you follow these four simple rules from the RetroAge Eating Basics, you will lose weight, have more energy and look and feel younger.

1. **Never drink liquids—even water—with meals.**
   Fluids dilute vital stomach acids that are necessary for digestion.
2. **Always include *raw* vegetables and/or salad with meals and raw fruit and/or juice between meals throughout the day.**
   Valuable enzymes found only in uncooked vegetables and fruit assist digestion and encourage new cell growth.
3. **Food Combine: Never combine animal proteins and starches at the same meal.**
   These foods must be eaten separately for proper breakdown and assimilation of nutrients.
4. **Systematically eliminate all Non-Foods from your diet.**
   After they all have been eliminated, there's still plenty of delicious food for you to eat!

Following these four simple rules, you can have all the delicious food you want and become more and more vital with each passing year. I follow this plan and my digestion is great and my metabolism is as active as that of a woman half my age! And, since I'm a vegetarian, it's easier for me. I simply avoid all animal products and eat till I'm satisfied.

I have boundless energy, am very slender—and totally satisfied. Finally. It can happen for you as well.

I wish I could give you a guarantee that you will *never* eat poorly again. The fact is that you probably will—almost everyone does from time to time. But I can promise that dedicated RetroAge Eating will help bring the systems of your body into balance, and this does wonders to remove cravings. In addition, you achieve extraordinary self-respect and discipline that will motivate you to keep eating better. Then when you do go off, you will be so sensitive to your body's needs that you'll know what you must do to get back on track again quickly, painlessly and, above all, free of guilt and shame—not to mention excess fat.

I must confess that there are rare times when those old cravings come up. No, they have not completely disappeared. Muffins and chocolate are my personal nemeses. What is so interesting is that each time I surrender to that siren's call and indulge in a gigantic blueberry banana muffin or a luscious bar of chocolate with almonds, it re-proves my theory: I gain weight, get tired, exercise less and, astonishingly, am hungrier!

Such cravings serve as a wake-up call for me to pay more attention to what I am eating, as well as to what I am doing and how I am feeling. Like inappropriate eating, depression, stress and inactivity can trigger imbalances and, consequently, tailspin eating. If you find that you are eating to allay stress, be aware of what you eat and make only healthy food choices. (If you've Blitzed your kitchen, you won't have anything but healthy foods on hand. Let's not kid ourselves: If it's in our kitchen, it'll end up in our mouths.)

You may have noticed that I haven't said a word about counting calories, computing fat grams or even portion sizes. This does not mean that I am not concerned with weight loss or that you will not lose weight. With RetroAge Eating, your body finds its own balance. I'm very careful about maintaining a lean, slender body. RetroAge Eating makes this possible. It has worked for me and for my clients and it will work for you too.

> **BEWARE: DON'T EVEN *THINK* OF RETRoAGE EATING AS A DIET!**
> *Diets are temporary, stopgap measures that set us up to fail.*

RetroAge Eating is a completely revolutionary style that you will follow for the rest of your life. If you faithfully abide by the principles explained in this chapter, you will reverse your destructive eating patterns, lose weight and gain health. As you provide your cells with youth-building nutrients, you will prove for yourself that it is truly possible to reverse aging, just as my clients have done through the years.

Who hasn't rationalized overeating in a restaurant with: "I have no control over what they serve, so I might as well give up and enjoy myself."

This is a perfect example of tailspin logic because you let yourself be pulled off track by rationalizing that you have no choice about how much you are served or how food is cooked in the restaurant. You're simply giving yourself a false excuse.

Here are some ways to get around this rationale so that you can stick to the program and still enjoy a night out:

- Request that the waiter not serve you water, and do not order a beverage. No exceptions.
- Ask the waiter to take away that tempting basket of white rolls and breadsticks and the little dish of butter. If you must have something to munch on while waiting for your meal, request a bowl of crudités.
- Don't even munch nutritious whole grain breads if you plan to have any animal protein with your meal.
- Stop eating halfway through your meal. Let your body decide whether you should finish the full serving or not. You can always ask for a doggie bag. If the servings are exceptionally large, you might even request a second plate, put half of your food on it and ask for *that* to be wrapped up before you start your meal.
- And, hardest of all: Skip dessert, coffee, tea and brandy. You *can* have fresh fruit one hour after eating, when much of your meal has been digested.
- Of course, resist the temptation to reward your good behavior with one of those free mints at the cash register!

AN APPLE A DAY . . . AND THEN SOME

> **THERE IS ABSOLUTELY NO WAY TO CREATE YOUTH WITHOUT SUPPLYING YOUR BODY WITH ABUNDANT NUTRIENTS.**

The American Cancer Society recommends that you have five fresh vegetables and fruits each day. With RetroAge Eating, shoot for *eight,* to supply the vital enzymes that keep the digestive process active and contribute to age reversal.

Don't let the number eight scare you. This is simpler than it sounds. For example, assorted fruit snacks between meals, large salads and cooked veggies as side dishes and soup with meals handily fill this nutritional quota.

Remember, you don't need *quantity*, you need *variety*.

Another suggestion: Instead of a mayonnaise-filled tuna salad sandwich, which is poor food combining, create a delicious all-vegetable sandwich of tomato, lettuce, avocado and sprouts tossed with vinaigrette dressing between two slices of whole-grain bread.

And don't forget freshly squeezed vegetable and fruit juices. They deliver a powerful shot of valuable nutrition! The operative word here is *freshly*. Drink juices as soon as they are squeezed or pressed. Time, light and temperature immediately begin to destroy valuable nutrients.

Even if you find yourself unable to totally eliminate Non-Foods, don't let a day pass without having eight of these health-giving foods. This gives your cells the raw material to create a youthful body, even when you slip.

ALTERING YOUR FOOD CONSCIOUSNESS

As you clean up the way you eat, you will also find your own attitudes and habits about foods altering. This was certainly true for me, and many of my clients have reported the same.

In the beginning, I cut back on red meats for health reasons. I soon felt "cleaner" and more energized, as my body thrived. I continued to eat poultry and seafood because they were lighter, less fatty and easier to digest. Then, a friend gave me a copy of John Robbin's most revealing book *Diet for a New America*, which profoundly altered not just my way of eating but my way of thinking. It took me ten more years to become 100 percent vegetarian: no eggs, cheese, milk or any other animal products whatsoever. Believe me, it wasn't easy. I have found the benefits to be so amazing that I came very close to making the last rule of RetroAging "Adopt vegetarianism."

My focus has shifted away from my own body's needs to the well-being of all life on Earth. I had never realized that animals were being brutalized to provide us with food. According to Dr. Michael Klaper, member of the board of advisors to EarthSave, 15 million animals are slaughtered each day to satisfy the American desire for meat. If we reduced our meat intake by a mere 10 percent, 100 million people could be fed using the land, water and energy that would be freed up from growing feed for livestock. This knowledge moved me deeply. I now believe that we should not harm or kill animals for our food supply—ever.

My friends and clients, Joy Pierson and Bart Potenza, owners of New York's Candle Cafe, are so committed to vegetarianism that they have adopted the motto "Be Kind to Animals, Don't Eat Them" for their restaurant.

I'm aware that this is an extremely complex and emotionally charged issue. We must find our own paths. It is not for me to preach vegetarianism, especially since it took me fifty-nine years to get there myself! Being a vegetarian has made a huge difference in my life, inspiring me to take even better care of myself and others.

AND WHAT ABOUT SUPPLEMENTS?

While I suggest that my clients take all-natural vitamins C and E and make certain that they know how to alter their diets for maximum nutritional benefits, I stop before recommending extensive supplemental therapy. Instead, I suggest that they consult health practitioners, nutritionists, books and magazines and health-conscious organizations to keep abreast of the latest developments. There is a wealth of information and products out there—from melatonin and bee pollen to free radical scavengers, DHEA, Pycogenal, Hydergine and various herbal concentrates. I suspect that many have real value, and if it appeals to you to explore these areas of age reversal, go for it! It's an exciting search.

Over the years I have experimented with everything from mega- to mini-doses as information evolved and became available. At this point in my life, I am able to sense my body's needs and supplement my diet accordingly. I feel best when I get the bulk of my nutrients from whole foods.

To satisfy your curiosity, but definitely not as a prescription, this is my personal daily regimen of all-natural supplements:

- 2 1,000 mg Bioflavinoid Complex Capsules
- 2 400 IU Natural Vitamin E Gel Caps
- 1 Calcium-Magnesium Tablet (1:2 ratio)
- 3 Pacific Sea Plasma Algae Tablets
- 2 Combination Conjugated Estrogen/Progesterone capsules
- 5 Antioxidant Free Radical Scavengers
- 1 Acidophilus Capsule
- 1 Garlic Capsule
- 20 drops of Oxygen Solution

For better or worse, this is what I'm taking now. One thing all my friends and clients know, everything about me is open for revision. As you can imagine, with all the new supplements and therapies surfacing, I am continually researching health, youth and the aging process for innovations. I love it when something challenging shows up to steer me in a whole new direction.

A note about vitamin C: Since ascorbic acid, particularly in time-release capsules, may be a strong irritant to the small intestines, I recommend using only bioflavinoids, which are natural and safe.

RETROAGE EATING IN A NUTSHELL

MEMORIZE THIS CHART FOR PROPER DIGESTION.
NEVER EAT FOODS FROM GROUP 1 WITH FOODS FROM GROUP 2.

Group 1: Starchy Complex Carbs and Vegetable Proteins

Rice, Wheat Barley and Other Grains, Corn, Tofu, Tempeh, Beans and Peas, Potatoes, Winter Squashes, Bread, Pasta, Chips, Pretzels, Cereals, Nuts, Seeds and Nut Butters

With starchy complex carbs and vegetable proteins, you can only eat vegetables and salad—in any quantity. Remember: Absolutely no animal protein, not even a splash of grated cheese, sour cream or yogurt.

Group 2: Animal Proteins

Chicken, Turkey, All Fowl, Fish (Canned and Fresh), Beef, Pork, Veal, Milk, Cheese, Yogurt, All Milk Products

When you eat proteins, you can only eat non-starchy vegetables and salad with them. Remember you must never have any starchy complex carbohydrate foods with your proteins.

ELIMINATE . . . SURELY, EVEN IF SLOWLY

All breaded and fried foods, including all non-baked chips. Note: "Organic" doesn't mean baked, or even healthy.

Combining different types of protein in one meal. (Cheese and meat, eggs and cheese, etc.)

All foods made with refined sugar, artificial sweeteners and artificial fat.

Fruit in combination with any other food. You may eat it a half hour before meals or one hour after meals.

Heavy intake of dairy products. (They're mucus-forming and contain animal fat.)

Sweetened and/or carbonated canned or bottled drinks, even those from the health food store. Fresh juice is healthy; these drinks are not.

Regular pizza. (Cheeseless with whole wheat crust is okay.)

All processed meats—Franks, Ham, Bacon, Sausages, Pepperoni, Pastrami, Smoked Fish, Lox. Anything with nitrates.

All refined flour and grain products. (Eat only whole grains).

Limit canned, bottled and frozen foods.

Hydrogenated oils, saturated fats.

Foods with chemical additives, coloring and preservatives.

Do not eat any dessert after a meal. Desserts are a fattening habit that will slow digestion and speed aging. You may eat fruit one hour after a meal.

THIS WAY OF EATING IS FOR YOUR ENTIRE LIFE. DON'T BECOME OBSESSED WITH HOW MUCH YOU EAT, OR WITH CALORIE COUNTING. PROPER WEIGHT CONTROL DEPENDS ON YOUR BEING SATISFIED AND NOT WALKING AROUND HUNGRY OR DEPENDING TOTALLY ON SELF-DISCIPLINE. IT WILL TAKE YOU TIME TO MASTER THESE ENTIRELY NEW CONCEPTS. THE BODY HOLDS ON TO OLD HABITS. SO DON'T BE ANGRY WITH YOURSELF FOR OCCASIONAL BINGES. A HEALTHY BODY CAN HANDLE THEM.

REMEMBER: KEEP IT SIMPLE!
The closer a food is to its natural form, the better it is for our bodies.

TIME TO BLITZ!

Now, with all the nuts and bolts of RetroAge Eating out of the way, it's time to begin your first kitchen Blitz. Notice I said *first*. As you become increasingly dedicated to reversing your aging, you'll find yourself Blitzing your kitchen—and everywhere else—at regular intervals. Besides, it's a great feeling to pare down your possessions—and your body.

We're going to empty your house of everything that doesn't aid you in achieving youth and well-being—starting with the kitchen. Use the RetroAge Eating guidelines to determine what to keep and what to toss. It's time to get out those garbage bags, put on your sweats and face all those "can't live withouts" that are cluttering up your kitchen.

Many times I have had a tug-of-war with a client over a box of macaroni or a bottle of ketchup. The client would prefer using it up, worrying about wasting a couple of dollars, rather than getting rid of what's wasting his or her youth. Think of this Blitz as throwing out your mistakes. You didn't know they weren't good for you when you bought them. Besides, worrying about money is definitely being penny wise and *age* foolish.

Here's a sample checklist for your first Kitchen Blitz.

KITCHEN BLITZ

Throw Aways	Possible Keepers	Keepers
Refrigerator		
Blue Cheese Dressing	Orange Marmalade	Cabbage
Mayonnaise	Low-Fat Mayonnaise	Romaine Lettuce
Sodas	Pasteurized	Dijon Mustard
(Including Diet)	Orange Juice	Snow Peas
Whole Cream/Half	Bottled Salsa	Yogurt (Live Culture)
& Half	Dill Pickles	Whole Grain Breads
Whole Milk	Free-Range Chicken	Almonds, Sunflower Seeds
Ketchup	Salmon Steaks	and other nuts
Hot Dogs/Bologna		Extra Virgin Olive Oil
		Roasted Sesame Oil
		Whole Grain Flour
		Steel-Cut Oatmeal
Cupboards		
White Flour	Granola	Fat-Free Rye Crackers
Bottled Spaghetti	Pasta/White Flour	Pasta/Whole Grain
Sauce (with sugar)	Water-Packed Tuna	Brown Rice
Packaged Macaroni	Canned Tomatoes	Barley
& Cheese	Packed in Puree	Dried Spices and Herbs
Canned Chili	Juice-Packed Fruit	Herbal Teas
Canned Ham		Green Tea
Canned Almost Anything		Dried Fruits

. . . You get the idea.

Now you're ready to make your own list. I suggest that you make several photocopies of this blank Blitz form, since you'll probably be Blitzing again and again once you get with the program! And don't forget to stock up on heavy-duty, super jumbo garbage bags. You'll be needing them.

KITCHEN BLITZ

DATE: _____

Throw Aways	Possible Keepers	Keepers
Refrigerator		
Cupboards		

4 STEP 2: EXERCISE

I always knew that I wanted the suppleness and endurance of a trained athlete or dancer who works out for hours each day; yet I also knew that I'm not the kind of person who has that much drive or self-discipline. For more than thirty-five years, I've been experimenting with ways to achieve extraordinary results in very little time, without pushing myself. I finally found my answer in a two-part plan. I call the first part Innercize because it involves sensing and visualizing my body in everyday activities. The second is a series of five simple exercises that keep me strong and flexible.

Since sensing and visualizing are mental activities, can they really affect the body?

It is known that when we simply think about a particular movement, the muscles involved in that movement contract. When we envision an action, the brain sends a movement message to the muscle sets. Now, I am not suggesting that you can run a marathon while reclining on your sofa. But, by visualizing muscle groups, you can learn to develop your body under diverse circumstances throughout your waking hours.

When physical labor was more a part of our routine—before industrialization—we naturally got sufficient exercise as an integral part of our daily lives. But as life got more mechanized, we moved less and, in our inactivity, our muscles became more flaccid. Today, to get adequate exercise, we actually have to choreograph movement into our lives. We buy exercise equipment, join gyms and actively seek ways to keep our bodies vital, strong and flexible. Paradoxically, it usually takes injury or illness to jolt us into beginning a regular exercise program.

In my case, since I've rarely been sick or injured, my motivation was to counteract the negative effects of aging. The techniques I will be sharing with you have helped me create a younger, more finely toned and flexible body and, along with RetroAge Eating, have kept my metabolism from slowing down. They also discourage those extra pounds from settling on my hips—their favorite resting place.

These simple techniques will help you form a new relationship with your body—a gentle, loving relationship. With Innercize, you carry a powerful mental image of your own skeleton and musculature. You will get to know your body intimately, making certain that you continually monitor and correct its movement for enhanced fitness and grace. I have found that when my clients realize that they truly can create the body they want, they become motivated to care for it in a way they never did before. They don't give up.

People have said to me, "Hattie, you've spent your life as a dance teacher. You've always been active. Is there hope for someone as out of shape and exhausted as me?"

My answer is a resounding "Yes."

Like most people, I have been through many stages in the course of my life. There were times in which I was too exhausted to be active. I have overeaten, been as much as twenty-five pounds overweight, carried two children, had cellulite, felt self-disgust. But I have come to bless all those experiences. They have shown me the magnificence of the body and its exquisite capacity for regeneration.

As you care for your body, you will develop a new respect for all that makes you a human being. And with that respect comes inspiration, glowing well-being and youth.

Before we move on, take yourself on a no-holds-barred guided tour of your body. Stand naked—or at least in your underwear—before a well-lit, full-length mirror. The three-sided kind you find in department store dressing rooms is ideal. Then fill out the How I View My Body Worksheet.

A word of caution: This mirror-and-notebook exercise may be very uncomfortable or even disturbing. That is not my intention. I merely want you to have a point of reference to gauge your progress. Don't be afraid to face yourself honestly and admit your fears and problems. The only way to change is to openly acknowledge what bothers you, and, rest assured, you will change.

Here's a client's sample to give you an idea of how specific, not to mention brutally honest, I want you to be.

HOW I VIEW MY BODY

What I Hate	What I Dislike	What I Like	What I Love	I Can Change
My hanging belly	Stretch marks on my stomach	My breasts	My complexion	My weight
My teeth and mouth	Scars on my legs	My dimples	My eyes and long lashes	Condition of my mouth
	My toenails	My hair color	Shape of my legs	Condition of my feet
	The calluses on my heels			

Remember to look at your *whole* body, without skipping any part. I often have to coach my clients to look at *all* of their body, from head to toe, back, front and sides. The woman who contributed this How I View My Body exercise for the book could look quite objectively at her image from the top of her head to her cleavage and from the top of her legs to her feet. She completely ignored her two-hundred-pound torso, with her pendulous belly, silvery stretch marks and distorted navel. In fact, the first time she filled in this chart she actually wrote "Everything" in the What I Hate column and "Eyes" and "Hair" in the Like column. With RetroAge, the What I Hate column shrunk and so did her torso!

What I'm asking you to do is look closely and *objectively* at your body, evaluate what you see and fill in the blanks. From this critical perspective, you'll be able to track your progress as you RetroAge.

In my case, I knew that if I wanted to have a young, toned body, I would have to face myself squarely, openly acknowledging parts of me that I would rather have ignored. The more I admitted my discontent, the more motivated I became, ultimately creating the body you see in my pictures. It was work, there's no denying that, but my body has become truly terrific. Yours can too.

HOW I VIEW MY BODY

What I Hate	What I Dislike	What I Like	What I Love	I Can Change

RETROAGE INNERCIZES—LOOKING INWARD

As important as having a clear-cut, realistic picture of our bodies is a clear sense of how we move them. That's where RetroAge Innercizes come in.

The first step to mastering Innercize is to take a walk—to the bookstore! Buy the *Anatomy Coloring Book* or any basic anatomy book that appeals to you. Study the chapters on the muscles and the bones until you have a clear sense how the human body is put together.

When you understand the musculature, skeleton and connective tissue and can actively envision how your body moves, you're ready to begin the following exercises. There are three parts to each:

- Observe
- Correct
- Imprint

DOING YOUR INNERCIZES

To transform your body, it is crucial that you do these Innercizes in front of a well-lighted full-length mirror.

First you will observe yourself as you normally sit, stand and walk. Then you will put in the corrections with *your eyes open* to study how your body looks as you alter your posture. Finally, you will repeat these corrections several times with your eyes closed, visualizing your corrected posture as you saw it in the mirror. With your eyes closed, you must rely on your memory to recreate these new sensations. This will indelibly imprint these newly corrected movements in your muscle memory.

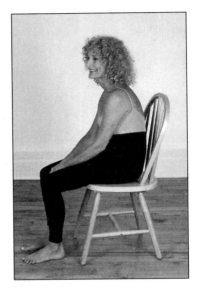

Observe

Pull up a chair and sit sideways in front of the mirror. Try to sit as you normally do. Here's what usually happens when people sit . . . Which ones happen to you?

Are you slumping?

Is your head tipped forward?

Is your stomach bulging?

Now that you have objectively observed how you sit, you are ready for the corrective exercises. Watch closely as you put in the corrections. If you're slumped over, notice how your body moves as you straighten your back and lift your head. Notice the sensation as you adjust your body and sit, balanced and upright, in your seat.

Correct

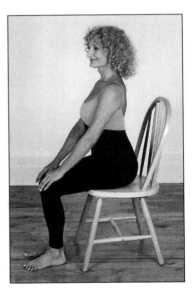

1. While looking in the mirror, slowly lift your spine, as if a string were pulling you up from the top of your head. Actually *experience* how your body feels. Sit forward almost on the edge of your seat, without your back contacting the back of the chair.
2. Keep lifting until you are sitting totally upright. This might feel uncomfortable at the beginning. We're so accustomed to slumping that this new, straight position may feel unnatural. Hold for a count of ten.
3. Slump again, then straighten up. Repeat this slumping and straightening process five times. At the end of the fifth time, hold the lifted, upright position for a count of ten. Once again, sense the feelings in your muscles as you put in the correction. Remember to keep breathing.

Imprint

1. Repeat Step Number 3 with your eyes closed. Picture your muscles as they lift your torso upward. In this way, you are imprinting your body with instructions to self-correct each time you sit, even when you're not thinking about your posture.

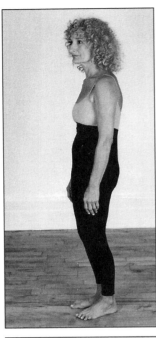

Observe

Stand sideways in front of the mirror. C'mon, don't suck in your gut! Stand as you normally do, not as you wish you did.

Are your knees locked?

Is your back hunched over?

Is your pelvis tipped back and stomach protruding?

Are your shoulders slumped? Are they hiked up?

Is your head tilting forward?

Correct

1. As you look in the mirror, start by tucking your pelvis under, tightening your buttocks and bending your knees slightly.
2. Lift your head and spine so that you feel an upward pull on your torso, as if you are suspended in midair, sensing an upward lift. Hold the corrected lifted position for the count of ten. Experience how your spine feels longer and your chest cavity more open.
3. Return to the slumped position, then straighten and slump five times. After the fifth time, hold the straight position for the count of ten. Keep breathing.

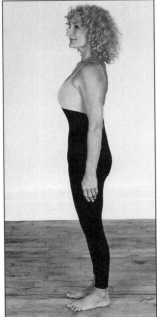

Imprint

1. With your eyes closed, repeat Step Number 3. Envision your muscles working to support you. This exercise will program you to stand properly automatically in your everyday activities.

You can also maximize muscle tone in your legs as you walk. It's difficult to use a mirror in your home to check your walk, so catch a glimpse of yourself in store windows, mirrors and other reflective surfaces as you walk along the street. What follows is what you should be striving for:

Observe

Are your head and jaw jutting forward?
Are you looking down at the ground?
Do you take small, cautious steps?
Are your arms stiff, as if you are afraid you might fall?
Do you like what you see?

Correct

1. Lead with your pelvis and take full strides, working your entire leg, from foot to buttocks.
2. Keep your chest, spine and head lifted. Take care that you don't jut your head forward.
3. Let your arms swing freely. Whenever possible, limit carrying things to a minimum. Women: If you carry a shoulder purse, cross the strap over your head to the opposite shoulder. Then relax both shoulders. And, if you use a backpack, use it *as* a backpack, on both shoulders.
4. Take your feet through a complete motion, first down on the heel and then following the motion through the sole and toes.
5. Keep breathing. It's amazing how often we hold our breath without realizing it.

Imprint

1. Since you'll bump into things if you walk around with your eyes closed, you must rely on your muscle memory to ensure that your corrections stay with you throughout the day.

**Do these exercises every day for two weeks
to reprogram your muscles.**

MAKING INNERCIZE PART OF YOUR LIFE

While sitting in your office, at the movies, watching television, whenever possible, check out your posture. Visualize your muscles as they lift and strengthen, just as they did in your exercises.

Do it now, as you're reading this. The more practice you have at sitting up straight, the more familiar it will become, until it becomes second nature. Remember how you looked in the mirror when you were slumping: shoulders sagging, ribs caved in, intestines compressed.

Notice the positive changes in your body as you lift: deeper breath, released pressure on your lower back, increased energy and a sense of exhilaration. Soon slumping will be the exception and not the rule.

Each day there are many times when we are just standing still, in an elevator, for example, or waiting in line. Use these downtimes as an opportunity to rejuvenate. Work on connecting and correcting as you did in your mirror exercises. Tighten your buttocks and abdomen, lift your rib cage, your spine, your head, breathe deeply. Imagine how the parts of your body are working. I have turned waiting time into mini-exercise sessions. No one knows that I'm working my pelvic and thigh muscles, tightening my stomach and lifting my spine while I'm waiting to cash a check or buy some fruit.

Throughout the day and during your routine activities you can create and reinforce your own well-being. Whenever you become aware that your body is droopy, slumping or tense, slow down or actually stop. Breathe deeply, lift yourself up and continue with your new muscle awareness.

From this point on, monitor yourself all through the day. Whenever you become unconscious of your body, aging takes over. Counter this with Innercize.

OCCUPATIONAL HAZARDS

Many professions have built-in perils. I've done body therapy sessions with clients—primarily lawyers, writers and musicians—who have lower back pain despite various forms of treatment. Most sit far too long, often in improper chairs that provide little support. When I've trained them to imagine their muscles lifting their spines, they improved their posture and relieved their pain. For dancers and athletes, problems are linked to overuse and injury. Incorporating Innercize into their exercise programs has uniformly helped them to heal rapidly and be less injury-prone.

Body consciousness is a major ally in the battle against aging. It will keep you young and connected to your being. Self-monitoring is a lifelong process. With Innercize you will view your body as the generator of its own youth and life force, and experience every moment as a new opportunity. You will carry a wonderful mental image of yourself as strong, sensational and ageless.

RETROAGE EXERCISES—BE FLEXIBLE FOREVER

The major difference between children's bodies and adults' is that children move with abandon. They bend and unbend effortlessly, fall and are not seriously injured. However, at about the age of twenty, the muscles start to tighten up and circulation begins to slow down. That creates a vicious cycle. When your joints are stiff, you move less. As a result, you become tighter and even less flexible. This in turn inhibits circulation—and around it goes.

RetroAge breaks this destructive loop.

Arthritis—the stiffening and inflammation of joints—is the second largest health problem in older people, second only to loss of hearing. Osteoarthritis affects 35 percent of the population by age thirty. Yes, thirty! It's shocking how quickly aging can degenerate the body. The RetroAge flexibility exercises work powerfully to prevent and alleviate some of the symptoms of arthritis and keep your body limber and pain free. Now you won't be a stiff before your time.

And, as if you need more convincing, exercise is also found to facilitate control of such potential killers as hypertension and diabetes and to combat bone-weakening osteoporosis.

The RetroAge Exercise Program may not be what you'd expect of someone whose favorite form of recreation is reggae dancing and who enjoys thumping her stomach with a medicine ball. These five exercises are specifically designed to increase flexibility. They will prepare your body for more aerobic programs, including sports, dancing and biking, as well as weight and strength training, as they appeal to you. When your body is ready, you'll find yourself gravitating toward more active exercise in a most natural way. I've done these exercises for years and they have kept my body limber and supple enough to do everything I've ever wanted to do.

Not everyone who begins the RetroAge program with me is able to execute these movements when they start. So, after the Actions for each, I have given you modifications to use until you acquire the agility to perform them perfectly. I have clients do these exercises once a day, preferably in the morning. Since they're so simple and take so little time, this is not a hardship. You'll be energized and clearheaded, getting your day off to a lively start.

Also, have you noticed that children always want to be touched and played with? Their bodies want to be touched and they reach out for it. Sadly, at some point in our growing-up process, we stop asking for what our bodies naturally crave. When exercising, be sure to touch and massage, and sometimes even pinch, pull and pound, your muscles. The power of touch keeps you young, and it keeps you mindful of how your muscles and joints are working.

RETROAGE EXERCISE BASICS

Stay mindful of these elementary rules for a successful RetroAging exercise program for fitness and flexibility.

- **Make sure you keep breathing throughout each exercise.**
  I'm serious. Most people hold their breath when they exercise. It's a good idea to sing, hum, count, sigh, grunt. Making sounds will remind you to keep breathing.
- **Never lock your knees or elbows.**
  When you tighten your joints, it cuts off circulation and puts pressure on the nerves and bones. You may feel stronger at the moment, but you end up weaker in the long run.
- **Don't arch your lower back.**
  We automatically pull up our lower backs when we strain, and when we're tired our backs arch on their own. Arching causes pressure on the discs and nerves, resulting in pain, back problems and a potbelly.
- **Keep your pelvis tilted forward.**
  This releases tension in the buttocks and legs and takes the strain off the lower back where most problems arise.
- **Do your RetroAge exercises daily.**
  Learn to enjoy the sensations in your muscles and joints as they become more limber and expressive.

Anti-Ager #1 ARM AND SHOULDER STRETCHES

Helps: Arms, shoulders, legs, spine, circulation and complexion.

Starting Position: Stand straight, legs slightly apart, toes forward and knees slightly bent. Sense the soles of your feet in contact with the floor and visualize your head and spine lifted.

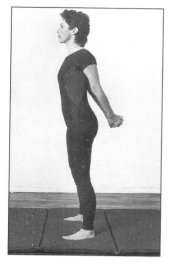

Actions:

1. Put your arms behind your back and clasp your fingers together.
2. Straighten your arms, pulling your shoulder blades together. Slowly and smoothly start bending forward, leading with the head.
3. Pull your clasped arms as far as you can upward, toward the ceiling. Hold for ten counts.
3. Slowly return to starting position, keeping the hands clasped firmly behind you throughout.
4. Repeat five times. Concentrate on bending lower each time.

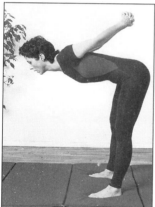

Reminder: Keep pelvis tipped forward and buttocks tight the whole time.

Alternative Actions: If you are unsteady on your feet or are unsure of your balance, sit on the side of your bed or on a stool. Sit evenly, with your legs parallel and relaxed. Then, put your arms behind your back and clasp your fingers together and proceed with the exercise as instructed.

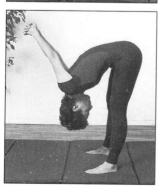

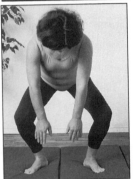

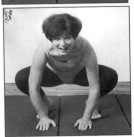

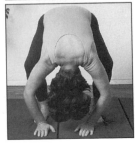

Anti-Ager #2 HIP AND KNEE BENDS

Helps: Feet, ankles, knees, hips, spine, neck, energy, speed.

Starting Position: Stand straight, legs hip width apart, toes pointed slighty outward, knees loose, not locked.

Actions:

1. With head down, slowly start bending your knees outward, reaching hands toward the floor.
2. Continue crouching, bending your knees outward. Lift head. Place palms on floor. Lift your heels, until you look like a frog ready to leap. Don't worry if you feel pressure on your toes and balls of your feet—this stimulation is good for them. Hold this position for a count of five.
3. With your palms still on the floor, lower head and torso and start straightening knees slowly and smoothly, while lowering your heels. Hold for a count of five.
4. Slowly lift torso and head and return to starting position.
5. Repeat five times. As you become more adept, hold #2 and #3 positions for a count of ten.

Alternative Actions: Again, sit on the edge of your bed. Balance your weight evenly on your buttocks. Spread your knees as far apart as is comfortable. Flex your feet and balance the weight of your legs on your toes. Lean forward between your legs, reaching your arms downward until your palms rest on the floor. Proceed as directed. Even though you're sitting, you'll still be working your knees and ankles.

Anti-Ager #3 SIDE TO SIDE STRETCHES

Helps: Hips, spine, midriff, arms, neck, lung capacity, endurance.

Starting Position: Sit on floor with right leg bent at knee in front and left leg to the back, knee bent. Distribute weight evenly on both hips. Hold head high and back straight.

Actions:

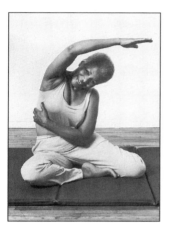

1. Reach up with your right arm while placing your left arm across your body to hold your right ribs.
2. Stretch your right arm way up, and bend to the left as far as you can. Imagine your arm tracing a large arc in the air. Pull your head sideways and down. Massage your ribs with your left hand.
3. Still holding your right arm upward, return to the starting position, continuing to stretch your arm in a graceful sweeping arc.
4. Reverse leg and arm positions and stretch to the other side.
5. Repeat five times to the right; five to the left.

Alternative Actions: If starting position is too difficult, extend leg to the side instead of bending it behind your body. If you are unable to get down on the floor or position your legs as directed, sit on the edge of your bed or on a sturdy chair and proceed with the upper body movements as directed. You'll still get the full benefit of the stretch.

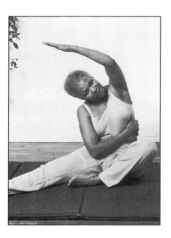

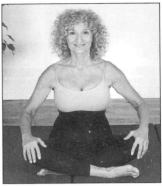

Anti-Ager #4 HEAD ROLLS

Helps: Neck, spine, relieves tension and stress.

Starting Position: Sit on the floor, cross-legged, hands on knees, elbows out, spine upright with head high.

Actions:

1. Slowly lower head to your left shoulder, leading with the very top of your scalp as if someone were pulling it with a string. Keep shoulders down. Massage right shoulder and neck with left hand to relieve tension.
2. Slowly lower your chin to your chest, then to the right side and finally to the back, emphasizing four points in space—side, back, other side, front. It may help to say, "Right, front, left, back."
4. Repeat five times then reverse the process: left, front, right and back.

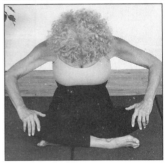

Alternative Actions: If you can't cross your legs, stretch them in front of you, spread as far apart as is comfortable for you. Make certain you're balanced and your weight is distributed evenly on your buttocks. You can do this sitting upright in a chair or on the side of your bed, or anywhere else you are sitting comfortably.

Caution: All movements should be slow and smooth, without jerking or forcing, especially when moving head to the back.

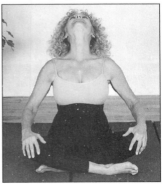

Anti-Ager #5 LEG LIFTS

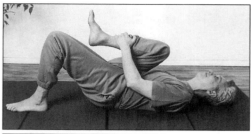

Helps: Lower back, abdomen, hips, ankles, legs, circulation.

Starting Position: Lie totally relaxed on your back, knees bent and feet flat on floor.

Actions:

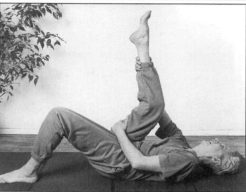

1. Lift right leg, knee bent. Clasp hands below your knee, on your shin if possible, and pull *gently* to your chest.
2. Clasp left arm behind your thigh. Place right hand on calf. Slowly straighten leg upward. *Do not pull.* Point toes.
3. When leg is straight as you can get it, alternate flexing your foot and pointing your toes five times.
4. Keeping leg extended, bring left hand to right ankle and gently ease leg backward. Flex foot to stretch hamstrings.
5. Lower leg, release your hands and return to floor.
6. Repeat with left leg.

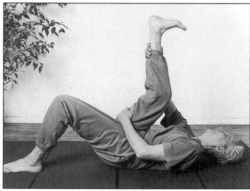

Alternative Actions: If you can't get on the floor, you can do this exercise on your bed. To avoid stress on your neck and shoulders, position a firm neck roll (or fashion one by rolling a bath towel) under your neck.

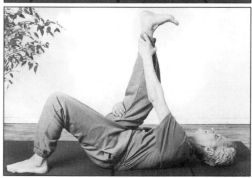

TIME TO BLITZ!

The Blitz associated with RetroAge Step 2 is the Wardrobe Blitz. By this time, you are more in tune with your body and how it works than ever before, perfect preparation for this Blitz.

So break out another box of garbage bags and put on your favorite CD and get to work.

Again, I suggest making several photocopies of this Wardrobe Blitz form for future use. I've never seen a client capable of conducting a complete Wardrobe Blitz at first attempt.

Just as you did when you Blitzed the kitchen, I want you to put everything in your closets and drawers into three piles. Your throwaway pile will contain all those old clothes from the back of your closet—you know, the outfits you'll fit into when you lose thirty pounds or that hold too many memories for you to part with. Well, I say, if you lose those thirty pounds, you deserve to buy something new. And who needs clothes to remember those special occasions when the memories are in your heart? If you use clothes to remind you of your youth, youth will remain in the back of the closet. RetroAge is about being young now and in the future.

Add to your throwaway pile all those clothes that make you feel and look old. Get rid of your polyester pull-on pants and those cotton housedresses. While you're at it, throw in those dowdy dresses that are "appropriate" for your age.

Now, I'm not saying you have to wear miniskirts and high heels (of course you can if that's what makes you feel good), but don't think that you have to dress a certain way because of your age. Wear what makes you feel good about yourself.

Possible keepers may include skirts you can shorten, items you can update with color and youthful accessories, and anything that you just can't bear to part with right now. (Remember, Blitzing is an ongoing process; what you can't get rid of today might be a throwaway tomorrow.)

Of course clothes that make you look and feel like a million bucks are keepers.

Once you Blitz, you'll probably have lots of room in your closet, so go out and buy something new. Don't be afraid to experiment. Go ahead, buy something daring and sexy. Or start slowly and add a colorful scarf or tie to your wardrobe. Remember the key is to feel good about how you look.

WARDROBE BLITZ

DATE: _____

THROWAWAYS	POSSIBLE KEEPERS	KEEPERS
Bureau: *(List by Drawer)*		
Closet #1		

WARDROBE BLITZ
(continued)

DATE: _____

THROWAWAYS	POSSIBLE KEEPERS	KEEPERS
Closet #2		
Basement/Attic		

5 STEP 3: SKIN CARE

NEW SKIN FOR OLD

For many of us, the only part of our skin that gets any attention is the part that shows. We take our morning showers, wash our face and hair and proceed to cover our bodies with the most flattering clothing we can find.

It's a shame too, since the skin not only covers and protects everything that makes up our physical bodies, it also is the largest organ in the body. It helps to regulate our body temperature and it serves as the outlet for an extraordinary amount of toxins. Now is the time to give it the special, loving care it deserves.

Of the four steps of RetroAging, skin care is my very favorite. For as many years as I can remember, I've taken great care of my skin, treating myself to luxurious massages and the finest aromatic natural oils and cologne I could find. This makes me feel clean and sweet smelling, and I love that!

People often tell me that I have young and beautiful skin. And I love that too. Now let's make sure you get your share of compliments.

There is no way you can be youthful without making sure that your skin is radiantly healthy. Exquisite skin is one of our most prized possessions. When your skin is beautiful, you feel beautiful. It doesn't matter what shape it's in to begin with. I promise you that consistent care will produce consistent results. Just don't give up—be relentless! It's worth it.

When was the last time someone said your skin was as soft as a baby's bottom? Recently, I hope, but I suspect that's not likely. With RetroAge Skin Care you will restore your body to its original silken smoothness—perhaps not precisely the aforementioned baby's bottom, but lovely nevertheless.

> **YOU'VE GOT TO GET ROUGH TO GET SMOOTH!**
> **Making old skin young is no gentle job.**

Be forewarned: The RetroAge Skin Care Instructions may appear odd at first, especially if you've always heard that you must treat your skin with kid gloves. My style leans more to boxing gloves! Don't worry. You're not alone in your doubts. Even my most dedicated clients were hesitant to try these techniques at first. Nobody had ever told them to brush their face with a dry brush before. Hair, yes, face, no. Or stretch and pull at the skin? "No," they protested. "It'll make it sag!" "I'll need a facelift!" Once they got over their initial shock, they never looked back. Several even decided against the face-lifts and eye lifts they were already planning.

THE BIG FOUR FOR SKIN CARE

Let's go over the four basic components of the RetroAge Skin Care Program:

- Exfoliation
- Circulation
- Hydration
- Detoxification

First we have *exfoliation*, the sloughing off of dead cells. Children's bodies are always growing and changing, constantly shedding skin cells.

Aging causes this process to slow down markedly, leaving you with unevenly textured, wrinkled skin. To keep youthful skin, you must help the process by *mechanically* exfoliating your entire body. Just as a carpenter sands a piece of wood, keep rubbing your skin carefully with rough cloths, brushes, pumice stones, gritty creams and soaps, and you'll be polishing your outer surface to a lovely glow.

This brisk removal of "old" cells unclogs pores and creates smooth, blemish-free skin, while encouraging new skin growth. Instead of leaving you rough and raw, you'll actually be lightening age spots, smoothing out imperfections and getting rid of callouses and other assorted unattractive "crusties" that time has managed to deposit on you. And it feels sensational too! I use sturdy natural fiber mitts and brushes for wet and dry exfoliation of my face and body every single day.

Dry brushing is an extremely powerful method for rapid exfoliation. Wet brushing is slower and gentler. Wet brushing can be done daily. If your skin is sensitive, adjust the frequency of dry brushing to avoid irritation.

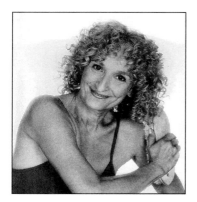

The first dry brushing I ever did was with a common, everyday scrub brush—like one you'd use on the floor—that I picked up in the supermarket for less than $3. Soon I had all of my clients scouring away. After a few weeks one regular client who had been seeing great results from her dry brushings reported that, to her horror, she returned home to find her housekeeper happily scrubbing away on her bathroom floor *using her precious dry brush*. So I recommend buying two—and hiding one for your exclusive skin care use.

Remember to scrub and oil your elbows. Wrinkly, dry elbows are a telltale sign of aging. I've even used fine-grain sandpaper to smooth them out. And make sure that your hands and feet are silky and soft. If you don't know how to give yourself a good manicure and pedicure, have it done professionally. Dry, dead cuticles and calluses, especially on the feet, are not only old-looking, they are also potentially painful. Anyone who's had sore feet knows what I mean: It's like you have a toothache all over your body.

Then there's *circulation*: the flow of blood through the veins, arteries and capillaries. That's how we get nutrients and oxygen to our cells, and get rid of impurities, wastes and toxins. Exfoliation provides surface stimulation, but we need exercise and deep massage to guarantee abundant blood flow to every part of our body, inside and out.

I believe we don't fully acknowledge the healing power of touch. Babies who are not cuddled and held are known to die. One can only imagine the effect the absence of touch has on us as adults. I haven't seen any statistics, but I suspect that the absence of loving touch accelerates aging. RetroAge changes that. The remedy for touch deprivation lies, quite literally, in your own hands.

The third component of skincare is *hydration*. Water, that precious fluid that carries youth-giving nutrients from our food into our tissues, is the single most important element in preventing cells from becoming dry and aged. The hydration process is achieved internally by drinking at least eight large glasses of the purest water available and eating a diet enriched with fresh raw fruits and vegetables. Externally, our skin is moistened through long baths followed by the application of emollient-rich oils and lotions.

Detoxification is the big bonus of the RetroAge skin care regimen. By mastering the first three elements—Exfoliation, Circulation and Hydration—you successfully rid your body of accumulated impurities,

---

RETROAGE SKIN CARE BASICS

Here are the four basic techniques of your daily RetroAge Skin Care Program.

- **Dry and Wet Brush** your *entire body*.
  Speeds up Mother Nature's exfoliation process for younger, smoother skin.

- **Massage** your muscles from head to toe.
  Increases circulation and vitalizes skin and muscle tone.

- **Drink** at least eight glasses of water each day.
  Maintains supple, dewy skin. Keeps it hydrated by drinking sufficient fluids.

- **Bathe** in a tub of warm water with moisturizing natural oils.
  Totally relaxes your body and relieves stress while cleansing the skin of youth-stealing toxins.

flushing away waste and poisons that have been locked in your cells. Once freed of these pollutants, your skin is radiant.

Skin is blessed with an astounding capacity to regenerate. Thankfully, there is no time in life that this process stops. Yes, it's true, aging may slow it down, but RetroAge skin care revs it up to childlike speed.

> **THE SKIN IS A FABULOUS INDICATOR OF HEALTH!**
> **Everything that is *wrong* with you**
> **ultimately shows up in your skin.**

If you're sick or under stress, your skin will appear dull and lifeless. You may also find that blemishes occur and your color becomes pale and ashen, blotchy or florid. If you have a cut that takes forever to heal, consult your health care provider. That is often a sign of serious illness, such as diabetes. When you are in good health, your skin radiates wellness.

Regardless of what you've been told, beauty is *never* just skin deep. I tell my clients that true beauty radiates from within. We all possess it, but first we must claim it.

WHAT IT TAKES TO HAVE GREAT SKIN

Has it ever occurred to you that the places our bodies wrinkle the most are the very ones we've been cautioned not to touch?

We women are constantly told to be careful with our faces, especially the delicate skin around our eyes. How often have we heard that we must never pick at blemishes, scrub vigorously or push and pull at our necks—or else. Can't you just hear your mother's voice right now?

And what about how men treat their faces? Compared to what we've been taught, men actually *abuse* their skin. They scrape their faces and necks with a razor every time they shave and, unless they're heavy smokers who spend every day of their lives in the sun, are none the worse for wear. In fact, they actually age a hell of a lot better than women do.

When I hit my forties, my neck started to look crepey. I might have been able to ignore this "predictable" sign of aging, but my then teenaged daughter, Rama, always eager to keep me on target, strode up to me, touched my neck, grimaced and groaned. Her not-so-subtle reminder made me realize I had better do something—fast.

I had already determined that I would never have cosmetic surgery —a decision I still hold—but I didn't like having this old-looking, wrinkly neck either. My body didn't look old—my skin from the neck down was still looking terrific. So why were my neck and face aging faster than the rest of my body?

I asked myself what was I doing below my shoulders that I was *not* doing from the shoulders up? The answer was clear: **I was making demands of my body.** I danced every day and did other athletic activities that stretched, pulled and moved every joint and sinew. I also made sure that I had weekly Aromatherapy massages to work out the kinks and relax me totally. I soaked in a hot tub for a half hour every day, vigorously rubbing and scrubbing my skin with a brush, loofah and pumice stone. The skin on my body and limbs looked and felt like a baby's— well, at least like the skin of a woman twenty years my junior.

Still, the skin on my neck and face looked dry and old. So I decided to experiment and began to include my face and neck in my rigorous daily workout. To my delight, the more I touched and creamed my skin, and the more I pinched, pressed and brushed my face, neck and chest the less crepey and more youthful they became.

Don't think I was lightly tapping with my fingertips or using feather-light strokes either. I was pinching hard enough for my skin to become pink and deeply enough to get to the fat and muscle tissue below. I even rubbed my eyelids and under my eyes *really* hard—a definite no-no, if you believe generations of "experts." I quickly learned that this increased circulation not only brought nutrients and oxygen to my muscles, but also helped to carry away the accumulated toxins and waste products. In short, I stopped being overly cautious. Now my face, neck and chest glow—and I look a considerably younger than my sixty years.

You can do this too.

LOTIONS, POTIONS AND MORE

Almost any face cream can make you *look* more youthful—temporarily.

What makes any skin care product work on a long-term basis is its application. It's the consistent *touching*, not just the product, that makes the difference.

While costly products may contain extraordinarily beneficial ingredients, using a relatively inexpensive product can also give you excellent results. Regardless of the price range or product, make certain that it contains no mineral oils or petroleum products, propyl or isopropyl alcohol as well as no artificial coloring or scents. These ingredients are potentially dangerous to the system. Absorbed by the skin, they are carried into the systems of the body where they have the potential of causing real damage.

The secret is to apply the product frequently enough—and with sufficient pressure—to stimulate the underlying facial muscles. Massage in small circles, pressing against the bone. Feel the pressure. It's not going to damage your skin, I promise.

In addition to massaging, pinch your skin. This will seem strange and even frightening to you at first. You're probably thinking, I can't do that. If I pull at my skin, it will stretch and sag. It might, if you pulled on the surface skin only, but what you are working on is the muscle and fat underneath the skin.

As you pinch and press, concentrate on the muscles and tissues close to the skull, imagining your skin lifting and toning. As you do this, you will increase blood flow to the muscles, nourish the skin and erase wrinkles.

One client shared this adorable chant with me: "I pull my skin every day. Winkles, wrinkles, go away." It works. Her skin is gorgeous.

Body muscles move the skeleton—arm muscles move the arm bones, leg muscles move the leg bones—but the facial muscles, with the exception of those around the jaw, don't move any bones. Eyelid muscles and cheek muscles aren't called upon to do hard work. Under-used muscles—wherever they are on the body—become flaccid and droopy.

I have learned that the more you work muscles, the healthier they become. This applies to the muscles of the face and neck as well as those of the buttocks and abdomen. Stretch and contort them; smile;

grimace, be animated. Unlike a balloon or a rubber band, facial muscles will not become permanently stretched out because, also unlike a balloon or a rubber band, they are living tissue nourished with food and oxygen, continuously regenerating and renewing.

I use a blend of natural essential oils to cleanse and moisturize my entire body. Along with dry and wet brushing, massage and luxurious, oil-rich baths, I do special facial exercises—you'll be learning them later in this chapter—and use the oils several times throughout the day.

ABOUT SKIN CARE

1. Do not use petroleum jelly, mineral oil, propyl alcohol, or any substances on the body that are not made of the finest, natural, non-chemical cruelty-free ingredients.
2. Don't be afraid to be rough with your skin. Elasticity increases as you stretch, pull and even pinch it. Take care to stay sensitive to your particular pain tolerance level, working deeply enough to energize your muscles and skin but not so hard as to cause bruising or injury.
3. Keep all your nails groomed, particularly on your feet, so bacteria and fungus don't take up permanent residence.
4. Pumice and scrape away all your calluses. If you ever develop a huge callus build-up, have them removed by a doctor or skilled manicurist. Don't let yourself grow a crust. Thickening of the skin is one of the more negative aspects of aging. Reverse it mechanically.
5. Have professional massages as often as your budget will allow—and take them as deeply as you can comfortably accept. The deeper the strokes, the more effectively they relieve stress.
6. Never use talcum powder. Instead, use cornstarch, which has no silicon in it. Talc can be horribly damaging on your skin.

AND WHAT ABOUT THE SUN?

In this age of holes in the earth's ozone layer, it is essential that we protect our skin from the sun. I'll not go into great detail about how dangerous extensive exposure to the sun's rays can be. You've heard it already. Instead, I'll simply ask if you want to your skin to look like a piece of thick, weathered cowhide. I don't. That's why I pay *a lot* of attention to my skin. Yes, I swim and play on the beach and even get tan. But I take protective measures that prevent damage. You can, too, provided you use appropriate protection.

Wear a hat with a wide brim or visor, especially when you're in direct sun. This will not only shade your eyes, but also protect your hair and scalp from drying. It is also imperative that you wear optically ground sunglasses with sufficient tint to filter out ultraviolet rays and glare. Sunglasses also prevent the formation of squint lines around your eyes.

Another word of caution: Avoid wearing perfumes, colognes or scented lotions when you will be exposed to the sun. These products, as well as such medications as antibiotics, birth control pills and hormone supplements, can cause horrible blotching.

I cannot stress this enough: Use a good sunscreen, regardless of the time of year, even when it's hazy and overcast. Whether you're a fair-haired, fair-skinned Viking or an ebony African Queen . . .

EVERYBODY NEEDS SUNSCREEN.

No matter what your skin color is, use the best *natural* sunscreen you can find, with a Sun Protection Factor of 25 to 30 on your face, 15 everywhere else. Apply it often, especially if you're in the water or if you're hot and sweaty.

Sunscreen will help to protect your skin from cancer, but it won't guard against aging. The only way to prevent leathery, damaged skin is to scrub and soak, scrub and soak, removing those wrinkle-forming layers of dead cells.

THE RETROAGE FACE-IT EXERCISES

Some of these exercises may appear weird, so you might want to start doing them in the privacy of your own bathroom with the door closed. No one will laugh at you then, and they certainly won't be laughing when they see the results! If you consistently perform these exercises, your face will look smoother and younger. I promise.

ABOUT RETROAGE FACE-IT EXERCISES*

1. Before you start, apply cream all over your face, making sure you lavish it around the eyes, lips and neck.
2. Do the following RetroAge Face-It Exercises while looking in the mirror to make sure you aren't creating any new wrinkles while you work.
3. Start with ten of each exercise and work toward doing twenty of each. Once you have learned to do them properly, you can do them any time, any place, without a mirror. When you're watching television is a good idea.
4. Do these exercises daily . . . if you can. If not, start with every other day. Once you see the results, you might decide to exercise your face as routinely as you brush your teeth.
5. Don't worry about overdoing it. Unlike motor muscles that carry your body from one place to another, these are not weight-bearers. They thrive with the workout.

EYELIDS

Reconsider that eye tuck you've been saving for. You may change your mind about surgery once you've mastered these lid-lifting techniques I call **Lid Lifters.** At first, you may be worried that pinching and pulling will make your skin sag. On the contrary, stimulation increases elasticity.

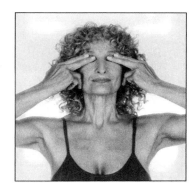

1. If you wear contact lenses, remove them before doing this exercise.
2. Pinch eyelids lightly with the thumb and forefinger, then rub and massage your entire lid with the pads of your fingers.
3. Make quick blinks in rapid succession, closing eyes firmly and then opening them wide. You'll probably notice that one eyelid is moving slower than the other. Concentrate on blinking both at the same rate. Start with twenty blinks and work up to a count of fifty. It's amazing how tired they get at first.

CHEEKS

My voice teacher pointed out that opera singers rarely have deep vertical crease lines between the nose and lips. In order to create those rich, round tones, they have to form the proper resonating chamber. They do this by pulling their lips forward and working their cheek muscles.

This exercise, which I call **Push-ups for the Cheeks,** will do the same for you.

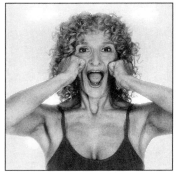

1. Stand up straight in front of the mirror, keeping your shoulders relaxed. Open your mouth wide.
2. Without closing your mouth, purse your lips, then relax. Press and contract your lips ten times. Relax and repeat three times.
3. Now firmly press the knuckles of each hand against each cheekbone and feel your muscles flex to iron out the lines. Pull your lips tightly inward, over your teeth

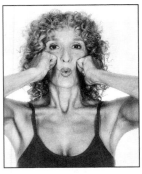

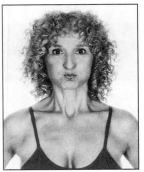

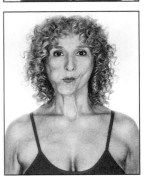

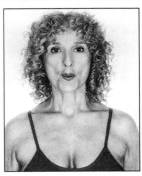

(as if pretending you have no teeth). As you do this, say "Ahh." Then press your lips together and say "Ooh." Alternate Ahh-ing and Ooh-ing ten times.

4. Do this exercise when you wash your face in the morning and at bedtime to discourage development of vertical creases between your nose and mouth, and to develop strong cheek muscles. You will feel this working the cheek muscles located inside your mouth.

Another of my favorite cheek exercises is called **Blow-Ups:**

1. Keeping your mouth firmly closed, blow up your cheeks in puffs, like inflating a tire with a pump. Hold for a count of ten; release.

A terrific way to soften your expression and remove wrinkles and frown lines around your mouth is the **Tongue in Cheek Exercise:**

1. Push your tongue firmly against each cheek and around your lips, pressing outward to stretch tight areas around the mouth and cheeks.

LIPS

Because of all the talking and eating we do in a lifetime, the muscles surrounding the lips carry a lot of tension—and get very little attention. One of the hallmarks of aging is the appearance of creases around the mouth and jaw. This exercise, **The Rubber Band,** will correct or prevent that problem.

1. Hold your mouth partly open with your forefingers, pull the corners apart as wide as possible, then quickly remove the fingers and let the mouth "snap" back to its relaxed position.
2. Open your mouth wide. With your thumb and forefinger, rapidly pinch and release the upper lip between your thumb

and forefinger. Work your way all around the upper and lower lips and cheeks.

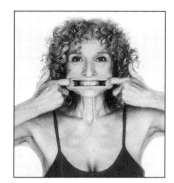

1. This exercise, **The Bugler,** mimics the way a trumpet player's lips are held.
   Blow hard, humming the sound "Brrr," making your lips vibrate.

TONGUE

The tongue, interestingly, happens to be the strongest muscle in the body. No one ever thinks of actually exercising it—other than when we talk or eat. Personally, I find this tongue exercise invigorating and fun. Besides, it does great things for the lips, chin and neckline.

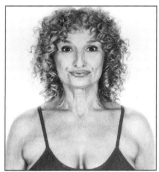

1. Open the mouth wide and stick your tongue out as far as it will go. Flatten and widen it and hold it there for the count of ten, then pull it back.
2. Lightly bite it at random.
3. Stick out your tongue and close your lips lightly around it. Then blow hard and make that obnoxious noise your mother told you not to.

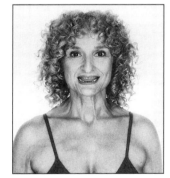

NECK

I suspect our necks age more quickly than our faces because we touch them less. In fact, we rarely even wash them unless we're taking a bath or shower. How often have you washed your face like it was a mask, stopping at your chin and hairline?

We may apply lotion every time we wash our hands, but ignore our poor necks. The next time you wash your face, note whether you automatically wash your neck as well; if you're like most people, you don't.

This exercise is not only good for your neck, it is also relaxing for your entire body. One word of caution: All neck exercises

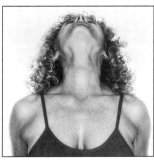

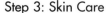

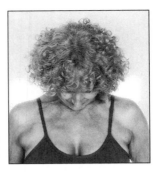

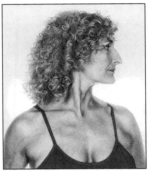

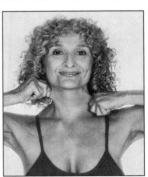

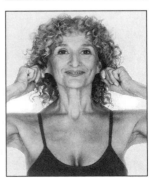

should be done slowly and without any force whatsoever, especially when you tilt your head backward.

1. Imagine that your head is a helium-filled balloon rising to the sky. With your back straight and shoulders relaxed, lift your head as high as you can.
2. Tilt your head slowly backward until it can go no farther. Keep your shoulders relaxed and down.
3. Slowly return to an upright position and then lower your chin forward until it touches your chest. Do not force it. Keep movements gentle and graceful.
4. Return to an upright position. Slowly turn your head as far as it can go from left to right. Resist the temptation to hunch up your shoulders to touch your chin. Keep shoulders down. Hold for a slow count of five, then move to the front, pause, then move to the opposite side.
5. Use your chin to "draw" the largest circle possible in the air. Remember to keep your shoulders down, lift your chin and slowly rotate first clockwise, then counterclockwise.
6. Hold your head erect. Grab the skin on your neck with your thumb and forefingers and pinch and pull it. This helps to get rid of that double chin.

EARLOBES

And what about those earlobes?

Earlobes?
Yes. Earlobes.

One common sign of aging that you may never have considered is droopy, dry earlobes. We rarely give them a second thought, but there they are, waiting to be touched. Give them a mini-workout by massaging them with a skin-softening lotion or oil. The results of this TLC will surprise you. You will erase one more unattractive telltale sign of aging—and it feels nice, too.

TO CUT OR NOT TO CUT

It upsets me to see people having face-lifts, tummy tucks and liposuction at younger and younger ages. Personally, I have vowed to never have any cosmetic surgery for any reason, barring a disfiguring accident. This decision is based on my reverence for nature and myself.

I am not alone in my decision to honor the changes that happen through time. I have been working with a former model who graced the covers of many high fashion magazines during her successful career. Now in her seventies, she is a glowing example of ageless beauty. She has never had cosmetic surgery and vows that she never will.

As she says, "There's beauty at every age. I don't want to look like a sixteen-year-old. Since working with you, Hattie, I feel like myself again. I feel beautiful."

I'm thrilled to have her as a client. Sometimes, when I feel discouraged about my aging, I look to her for inspiration.

ONE MORE THOUGHT

Each day, when you brush your teeth, also brush the insides of your cheeks, your tongue and the roof of your mouth. When the inside's healthy and clean, it shows on the outside.

The Blitz assigned to Step 3: Skin Care is, quite appropriately, the Bathroom Blitz. Throw away *every* tube, vial, jar and bottle of every skin care, hair care and makeup product that doesn't contribute to your regeneration. Also use this as an opportunity to discard every past-dated prescription drug and over-the-counter medication in your medicine cabinet.

It's certainly time to throw away the frosted blue eye shadow and bubble-gum pink lipstick. In fact, all old makeup should be discarded, as bacteria can form and cause infections. Eye shadows shouldn't be kept for more than six months. The same goes for lipstick. As for mascara, toss it after three months.

You may be reluctant to surrender your petroleum jelly and baby oil as well as all those products that contain alcohol, coal tars and synthetic colors—including hair products, cleansers and certain makeup. You certainly may hold on to them for now. Hopefully, by the time you do your next Blitz, you will have decided to use only natural products in caring for your skin.

Natural essential oils, a good-quality moisturizer and a natural sunscreen with an SPF of at least 15 are definite keepers.

Treat yourself to some new makeup. Go to the cosmetics counter at a local department store and ask the saleswoman for some help. You usually can get a free makeup application. Even if you don't buy, it's a great way to experiment with new colors and looks.

Blitzing your bathroom is a great way to keep your skin care regimen on track and keep your bathroom free of clutter. So get out your garbage bags, put on your favorite CD, light a few scented candles, and get to work! Again, I suggest photocopying the Blitz form for future use. I have clients who blitz every couple of months. I do.

BATHROOM BLITZ

DATE: _____

Throwaways	Possible Keepers	Keepers
Medicine Cabinet		
Vanity		

6 STEP 4: ATTITUDE

CHANGE YOUR THINKING, REVERSE YOUR AGING

Peter Pan had a point. Who in their right mind would want to grow up if growing up means getting decrepit?

I believe that people who age badly have bought the image of the doddering old man or the little old lady with a walker. Our mental images play a huge role in controlling how we age. If you expect to become incapacitated, incompetent, with wrinkled, sagging skin, it'll probably happen.

Well, here we are at Step 4: Attitude.

While all four steps of RetroAging are vital for looking and feeling younger, I am tempted to say that this step is the most important. Attitude is a powerful component of the RetroAging Program. Unless the mind is steadfast in its positive focus, age reversal is a pipe dream.

In our society we are programmed to age poorly. Notice how often the media reinforce a pathetic view of aging, especially with women. As you can imagine, this never sat well with me.

In developing this program, I often questioned why age has become so abhorrent in our culture. We have been brainwashed by so many distorted thoughts about growing older that, rather than welcome aging, we resist it—and you know what resistance does! It helps build a critical mass of fear and creates still more resistance. We lose even before we begin.

For many of us, the passage of years is dreaded and feared, while youth is viewed with favor. And it's not just society that's handing us this deadly scenario, it's our own minds. These preset concepts—many formulated in childhood—sabotage almost half of our lives. We don't even give ourselves an opportunity to try our hand at what's possible as we live longer.

Not only is this unfortunate, it is dangerous. The mind is an awesome force, as we have all experienced. When it delivers destructive images, they are well on their way to becoming true. Thankfully, the reverse is equally true. We *can* reprogram ourselves to become younger in ways far more powerful than a mere "You're only as young as you think."

However, before we can begin RetroAging Step 4, we must first identify what we actually think about aging. So get to work on your How I View My Aging Worksheet.

An overstressed, underenergized woman in her mid-fifties had written off a series of physical changes and personal experiences as inevitabilities of aging. In the process of filling in the blanks of this exercise, she altered her thinking, as well as her activity level and saw that (1) the stiffness in her knees and fingers could be easily alleviated with a simple stretching program; (2) her fuzzy vision could be corrected by *weakening* the prescription in her eyeglasses, and (3) she could still tap dance.

"I was turning into an old lady before my very eyes before I began RetroAging. Now my life is an adventure and my body is up to the excitement my future holds," she explains with a smile.

Here's a sample of her How I View My Aging exercise for inspiration.

HOW I VIEW MY AGING

Ways That I Am Old	How That Makes Me Feel	Ways That I Am Young	How This Makes Me Feel
My knees and hands are stiff when I wake up in the morning.	Old and cranky. I'm okay if I stretch before I start my day.	I love to dance, especially tap, and I'm still good at it.	Sassy . . . like a kid again.
I have no patience for loud children in restaurants and their parents who let them misbehave.	Like my grandmother.	I still love rock and roll.	Twenty . . . but it makes me feel weird when I hear deejays and young adults call the music of my high school and college years classic or nostalgia.
I'm afraid I'm going to die alone, a lonely old lady with her cats and flowers. I never felt this way when I was younger.	I've seen a lot of these old women living in walk-ups in my neighborhood. Some are vibrant and alive; others are bitter and mean. In my book, misery is optional.		

Now that you have the idea, have a go at it.

HOW I VIEW MY AGING

Write down ways that you consider yourself to be old followed by ways that you see yourself to be young and then openly admit how this makes you feel.

Ways That I Am Old	How That Makes Me Feel	Ways That I Am Young	How This Makes Me Feel

With Innercize you imprinted your muscles with new, powerful images and actions. Now you will put a different message into your mind—a positive RetroAger—to completely alter your thinking, and consequently your feelings, about aging. This harnesses the strength of negativity and turns it around, focusing on the pluses and canceling out the minuses. I call this Transforming Your Negative Aging Voice.

The more you practice, the more capable and confident you'll become. Regrettably, thinking positively about ourselves has been trained out of us. We must retrain ourselves to appreciate and love the person that we are. With this self-acceptance comes newfound strength and beauty. I sometimes imagine that I'm my own child. How would I treat me? Much, much more lovingly. So I switch my way of being and become more patient, affirming and caring. It works wonders.

At first, you may believe as I once did, that it's not possible to reverse aging. You may be attached to the inbred idea that aging goes only one way—downhill. RetroAge teaches you that this is not so. The body, mind and spirit are blessed with an infinite capacity to transform and regenerate, consequently growing younger.

With this exercise, you are urged to uncover your conditioned negative belief system around aging. Perhaps you'll be amazed at how angry and even repulsed you are at the prospect of being old. It was only after I openly admitted my fears that I was able to counter this pervasive negativity.

Believe me, Transforming Your Negative Aging Voice is not easy. It takes a lot of hard work. I would say that this mental exercise is a lot more difficult than any physical challenge. These negative messages about aging are deeply entrenched. We have been accepting these images all our lives; getting rid of them will not happen overnight.

TRANSFORMING YOUR NEGATIVE AGING VOICE

Examine your own recurring negative thoughts that you have about aging—your Negative Aging Voice. Rewrite each in a positive way, contradicting the negative notion with a rich, rewarding picture. This is your RetroAger. Here are some examples to get you started:

Negative Aging Voice	*RetroAger*
* Aging is inevitable. No matter what I do, I will become weaker and less attractive as the years go by.	* I control my own aging process completely. As I transform my thinking, I become stronger and more attractive with each passing year.
* It is not appropriate for me to wear revealing, sexy clothing. That's only for the younger generation.	* I have always loved wearing sexy clothes and will continue to wear whatever makes me feel beautiful—no matter what anyone thinks or says.
* Old people have old, ugly, dry skin, no matter what they do. I'd better start saving for a face-lift.	* My skin responds so beautifully to what I give it that I'll never need cosmetic surgery.

TRANSFORMING YOUR NEGATIVE AGING VOICE

Now list *at least* ten negative aging thoughts that keep popping up in your mind. Don't hold back. Get down and dirty with yourself. Don't rule anything out, no matter how insignificant it initially seems. *Work on this list at least ten minutes a day* until you are clear about your thoughts and have covered every area of your life. Refine your RetroAgers until each one is a positive, *bold* statement that powerfully contradicts the nagging negative.

NEGATIVE AGING VOICE	RETROAGER
1._____	1._____
2._____	2._____
3._____	3._____
4._____	4._____
5._____	5._____
6._____	6._____
7._____	7._____
8._____	8._____
9._____	9._____
10._____	10._____

When I first started transforming my negative aging voice, there were many occasions when I slipped back into that old mode of thinking. But as hard as this process is, I decided that, no matter what my mind or society's unsupportive stance brought up, I would stay focused and **GROW YOUNGER WITH EACH PASSING YEAR.**

Yes, I said *grow younger.* This may sound absurd. I certainly agree that it's an unusual statement, but I had made up my mind to marshal all my resources and transform aging, not only for myself and my clients, but for everyone else who found this prospect appealing.

My background as a teacher of dance gave me a unique head start. For more than twenty years I taught creative dance to hundreds of preschoolers. The memories of my students as they ran, jumped, fell, giggled and jostled one another remain with me to this day, an ongoing source of what it's like to be young, and I mean truly young—like a child. The greatest lesson they taught me is

IT ALL HAS TO DO WITH SPIRIT . . . AND SPIRIT IS AGELESS.

With this understanding to inspire and nurture me, it was no big deal. When my hair started to turn gray and my skin to wrinkle a bit, I did not panic. These superficial aspects of aging felt less significant to me. Don't get me wrong. I didn't give up on my appearance when these harbingers of age arrived. I simply dealt with them, intensifying my practice of all four steps in my personal RetroAge program.

Though beauty and glamour remained very important to me, I drew on my spirit, energy and heightened self-respect for power. In short, I experienced a deep shift in my attitude: I no longer dreaded the prospect of aging. From deep within, I knew that I had the capacity to take aging into my own hands.

The shift happened on the inside, but the transformation was showing on the outside. I was visibly looking younger. My stamina soared. I became stronger, more creative, courageous . . . lighter. Not only did I lose weight, I lost the heavy burden of worry and fear as well.

I no longer dressed, moved, behaved or thought like the stereotypical older woman. Whenever I detected any "old lady" behavior, I consciously put in an *immediate* correction. Similarly, when thoughts like "Oh, I'm too old to do that" or "Why would a young man like him be attracted to me?" came up, I listened without buying into that debilitating conversation. I may not have been able to stop my mind from thinking these thoughts, but I certainly didn't plan to allow them to overrun my life.

Each time they showed up, I used the technique of Transforming Your Negative Aging Voice.

When my clients, many of whom also anticipated losing their youthful energy, sexuality and vibrancy as they grew older, started transforming their own negative aging voices, they too become glowing examples of agelessness.

One client, a successful astrologer, now in her early sixties, relates: "When I first met Hattie, she was so energetic that I could hardly believe we were almost the same age. Now I'm about as young as she is. Her wonderful support in acknowledging me and helping me to change destructive thinking habits has transformed my life. I find RetroAging to be a continuing source of encouragement to live a vital life. It gives me practical solutions to aging problems and a new look at my possibilities."

This woman now eats properly and takes long walks. Her practice is thriving and she has finally begun to write a long-desired book about astrology.

She is not a rarity.

RetroAge gives you the power to decide exactly how you want to age.

Yes, it's true. You may not have precisely the same skin or muscle tone you once had, but you won't let that stop you from growing younger each day. For true youth is vibrancy, energy, courage, joyfulness and openness. And we never lose our innate ability to generate these qualities for ourselves.

As you complete the worksheets in this chapter, allow your mind to really let go. Listen to your thoughts and respect them, even if they are depressing or discouraging. Don't be fearful of negative thoughts. This will give you valuable practice in turning them around, and, I assure you, it takes practice. Be patient with yourself.

When people ask, "How long does it take to RetroAge?" I answer, "Your whole life—if you're lucky."

ALTERING ATTITUDES ABOUT AGING

Traditional Concepts	RetroAge Ideas
Be careful, cautious and gentle. You become more fragile as you age.	Don't overprotect yourself. The more active you are, the healthier, less injury-prone you are.
Expect to have aches and pains to limit your activities when you're old.	There's no need for aches and pains to stop you from *anything* unless you are not well. If you work at it, you will be fit at any age.
Expect to lose your marbles when you reach a certain age.	Aging doesn't stop learning, inactivity does. When you keep challenging your mind, it will stay clear, focused and developed.
Sex drive diminishes with age.	Sex becomes more intimate and fascinating as you mature.
Old people should act their age. Be dignified and appropriate.	Stay young by allowing yourself to laugh, be silly, have fun and play. Joy is not just for children.
Possibilities diminish with age. Rein in your goals.	Be unstoppable. Now that you have a few years behind you, you have the wisdom *and* the time to do all those things you dreamed of as a youth.
Old people know how hard life is and worry a lot.	Everybody, regardless of their age, worries. The trick is to stay in action. Life's hard enough without making up things to fret over.
You can't fight Mother Nature.	Why not? It's good exercise.
After forty, you're over the hill.	Keep climbing and you're never over the hill.
Now add some of your own:	

At the beginning the downsides seem to prevail, but soon you'll become skilled at rapidly contradicting the entrenched Traditional Concepts, replacing them with positive, inspiring RetroAge Ideas. Don't worry if you feel depressed, disgusted, discouraged. It takes time to change old habits and destructive ways of thinking. *Rome wasn't destroyed in a day.*

LET THE CHILD IN YOU SPEAK

As I see it, one of the most enchanting characteristics of children is their candor. When I was teaching dance and movement to preschoolers, not to mention when my own son and daughter were small, I was fascinated by their free-spirited, freely expressed opinions. If they liked something, they said so; if they didn't, they told me what they thought in no uncertain terms. They giggled, guffawed, laughed till they fell down. They stuck their tongues out at each other, and at convention. They were children, fully expressed.

As we age, we socialize and, of necessity, learn to curtail the expression of our feelings. Did you ever hear your parents say, "Big girls don't say that" or "You're too grown up to cry, son"? Unfortunately, as we learn these so-called "adult" manners, we also learn to lie. We learn to refrain from saying what we see, think and feel, lest we hurt someone's feelings or cause embarrassment. These withheld sentiments hold us back and make us inflexible.

The more you hold back, the older you get. As far as I'm concerned:

TRUTH = YOUTH

If your friends *really* knew what you thought—especially about them—would they still be your friends? And if they would think less of you for being honest, are they really your friends? And do you really want them for friends if you have to be constantly on your toes, taking care of their feelings? How can you be relaxed and fully self-expressed when you're always on your guard, weighing every thought that comes into your head or word that comes out of your mouth?

Can you imagine how great it would be if everything you said could simply be heard—without rage, resentment or hurt feelings? You'd be amazed at the amount of humor this releases. Try it, starting with your closest friends. Pretty soon you'll be playfully teasing each other with words that would have fractured your friendship in the past. You should hear Sallie, my co-author, and me when we get going—when she calls me a wrinkled old witch and I get back at her by calling her a fat no talent. We end up laughing and hugging each other. And what about Regis and Kathie Lee? They tease and chide each other all the time, and when I was on their show I saw that they were the best of friends.

Insulting yourself works wonders too. The final worksheet in this chapter opens the door for two-way free expression so that you actually learn to *love* criticism. It works this way: If you can acknowledge criticism, and anything else about yourself that may be perceived as negative and ugly, *nothing anyone else says can hurt you, because it won't be anything you haven't already said for, and to, yourself.*

This unbridled candor may not be your cup of tea at the beginning, but after you get over the initial shock, it becomes freeing. What could be more liberating than facing your own demons and neutralizing them?

My only request is that you be totally truthful with yourself. Say those horrible things that would absolutely wound your very soul were someone else to address them to you. Tell your "ugly" little secrets. That takes the sting out of them.

Remember: Free and open expression is one of life's greatest joys. With it, everything lightens up. You'll soon discover the relief of not holding back your thoughts and feelings. With this permission to openly express truth, the natural affection behind anger, fear and judgment bubbles up, leaving a wake of intimacy and love. Here's your personal Insult Sheet to fill out. I hope you enjoy the experience. I absolutely love it.

INSULT SHEET

Don't hold back. Be crude and even vulgar if necessary. Then rate your insults from 1 to 10, with 1 being a mild sting and 10 being a major ouch.

10 TERRIBLE THINGS THAT CAN BE SAID ABOUT ME NOTE: Make sure you pick things that could "hurt your feelings."	RATING
1.	
2.	
3.	
4.	
5.	
6.	
7.	
8.	
9.	
10.	

When I ask my clients to do this exercise, I have them read their answers to me. By the time they are through, they're in tears—of laughter! Miraculously, this Insult Sheet takes the weight off of these deep dark secrets, disempowering their seriousness and their hold over you.

HATTIETUDES BUILD HAPPINESS

Identifying our faults and foibles and poking fun at our negative ideas about our bodies, and aging in general, are powerful tools in our RetroAge kit. However, life is full of times that sadden us, shock us, bring us to our knees. Sometimes we need an inspirational nudge to keep our spirits up and alive. For this purpose I have developed a technique that I call *Hattietudes*.

We know that our words are powerful. Hearts can be broken by a syllable; enterprises launched by a simple, declarative sentence. My clients and I are living proof that you can talk yourself into reversing aging.

So, you ask, what *are* Hattietudes?

Hattietudes are positive statements that exercise a potent, affirming quality. They are designed to motivate our entire beings and counteract those negative forces that hold us back. They are ideas that jar us into consciousness. They are "booster shots" to inject us with new energy.

A professional woman who was new to RetroAging said, "I thought Hattie was just another rah-rah, personal empowerment type until I started reading her list of Hattietudes while I was waiting to be interviewed for a new job. I was anxious and almost sure that I'd be passed over for a younger person. In a few minutes, a sense of powerful calm settled through my body and I began to relax and feel more confident. I went in and absolutely nailed the interview, and ended up with a position a level above the initial job I was seeking."

I encourage my clients to tack their Hattietudes list onto the wall beside their desks, on their refrigerator doors, and on their bathroom mirrors, and to put it in their daily planner—places where they can see the list throughout the day and get a little boost from time to time. The following 20 Hattietudes to Inspire You to RetroAge are a jumping-off point for many more powerful personal statements that you can develop for yourself.

20 HATTIETUDES TO INSPIRE YOU TO RETRoAGE

1. Age is not the reason, it's the excuse.
2. Never forget the *You* in Youth.
3. Impossible = I'm Possible
4. Life may get harder, but you get smarter.
5. The hands of time are yours. Take aging into your own hands.
6. Don't let gravity get you down.
7. Fighting Mother Nature is good exercise.
8. Love is contagious. Go out and catch some.
9. Your first youth is a gift of nature; your second is a gift from yourself.
10. Convert envy into inspiration and you'll never run out of fuel.
11. Blame and shame maim.
12. Age doesn't make you forget . . . it teaches you what's important to remember.
13. Bless every rejection. It takes *hundreds* to get one good yes.
14. Wrinkles don't make you old. Babies have plenty of them.
15. Suffering is an option you don't have to pick up.
16. Where there's a will there's a won't. Respect the negative.
17. Never give up your dreams. They keep you awake.
18. If it's been done, you can do it. If it hasn't, you can be the first.
19. Learn to love hard work. It's the only way anything gets done.
20. Youth isn't wasted on the young—or on anyone else!

My clients have shared some of their personal Hattietudes with me so that I can pass them along to you.

- I can now treat myself exquisitely, no matter how others have treated me and how I have treated myself in the past.
- I will find my own personal style of experiencing aging so that I am excited at what the future holds.

- I can change my negative habits of behavior and thought into positive, life-affirming actions.
- It is a privilege to share myself with others.
- I am truly grateful to be alive—at any age.

The secret is to formulate statements that resonate to your own sense of self, statements that add fire to your spirit.

ABOUT ATTITUDE

1. Don't expect your attitudes towards aging—and yourself—to change overnight.
2. Don't allow backslides to discourage you. Backslides are to be expected. Keep working in the face of them.
3. Don't think you are too old for really dramatic changes.
4. Consider that what you think about aging is based on your past history, and the past history of humanity (in our culture). It may be entirely off the mark and ready for major revision—culturally and personally.
5. BE READY TO GIVE UP OLD CONCEPTS, HABITS AND POSSESSIONS.

   BE PREPARED TO GET DEPRESSED, DISGUSTED, DISCOURAGED!

   REMEMBER THAT THE FIRST STEP TO TRANSFORMATION IS DISCONTENT AND DISGUST WITH WHAT ALREADY EXISTS. I CALL THIS "CREATIVE SELF-DISGUST."

TIME TO BLITZ!

I call this the Everything Else Blitz because, as a grand finale to your RetroAge program, you rid your life of any clutter that remains. By periodically phasing out things that you neither need nor use, you are able to soar! There's nothing holding you back.

Break this Everything Else Blitz into manageable segments so that you don't become so overwhelmed that you throw in the towel. This is a highly personal, subjective process. If a picture of you as a lanky, freckle-faced nine-year-old boy in a cowboy outfit sitting atop a giant horse at the state fair many years ago brings back fond memories of joyful times and inspires you to stay in touch with that child's energy and spirit, don't even think of tossing it. In fact, you may even want to frame a blowup for your desk or assemble an album of such pictures and souvenirs that make you happy.

On the other hand, if you honestly have no feelings one way or the other or, if some bring up distressing, upsetting memories, get rid of them. Offer them to your aunt who keeps track of your family's genealogy or your cousin George who was hanging on behind you on the back of that horse. Send them to friends and family members who are pictured, with a short thinking-of-you note or rip them up and throw them out. Just don't stuff them back into that shoe box and put it back on the top shelf in the hall closet.

Personally, I would evict from my home all reading material but my dictionary, thesaurus, telephone directory, film and videoguide and whatever book I am currently reading. Any reference material and recreational reading can come from my public library. However, many people value the books on their shelves as highly as the gold in Fort Knox. Others, however, buy a book, read it and stuff it on a shelf, never to think of it again. When you blitz your bookshelves, decide where you are on this spectrum and work from there. Then organize the books that you do keep in an attractive, accessible way on your shelves. You can call Goodwill or your favorite thrift shop and donate the rest—or give them to your neighborhood library or sell them to a used bookstore. Just Blitz them out of your way.

Go into your attic and ask yourself if you really need the cribs and high chairs your now-grown children used; the dresses you—or your kids—wore to proms decades ago; old suits; broken radios and appliances you never repaired—and everything else you can find. Ask why you're holding on to these things. Do they serve a positive purpose in your life? If you can't just throw them away, ask yourself, Is there someone who could really use these things? Then give them away quickly.

Now take ten deep breaths and move on to your basement and garage and do the same thing. Get rid of all the things that clutter your life, make you feel bad or keep you trapped in the past. Remember that you're clearing the way so you can be fully alive in the present.

One final reminder: Just make sure that you have enough jumbo garbage bags and heavy-duty garbage cans within easy reach. Enroll a buddy to help you with the really big jobs, and, if you are moving out boxes of books or old clothes and appliances, arrange in advance for them to be carted away the day you Blitz. More throwaways than you can imagine have found their way back onto a closet shelf or into a freshly Blitzed basement simply because they were waiting for a pickup.

EVERYTHING ELSE BLITZ

(Use these forms for closets, basements, attics and other storage areas)
Photocopy as necessary

DATE _____

THROWAWAYS	POSSIBLE KEEPERS	KEEPERS

7 OWNING YOUR YOUTH POWER

I thought that I was just trying to look younger and sexier, but my personal RetroAging delivered me an unexpected bonus. I have watched myself transform from an often frightened, sometimes foolish, less than courageous "older woman" into a glowing example of personal integrity and inspiration.

Once I too viewed aging as a living death, but decline and decay were not what I envisioned as the perfect way to spend the second half of my life. Fortunately, rather than paralyzing me, my fears of aging propelled me into a lifelong search to avoid what I deemed inevitable. I have never been so glad to be proven wrong.

My youth quest has gone far beyond my original goals. It has brought me to a life of radiant health, dignity and the capacity to continuously generate compassion and joy in the face of anything that life delivers.

Now that you are experiencing the positive effects of RetroAging, you will notice what wonderful coincidences keep happening all around you. Opportunities for work, for relationships, for play, simply *show up*.

These seemingly chance occurrences are not serendipity. Instead, they are reminders that you are on target. Suddenly you will find yourself resurrecting dreams that you abandoned years before as unattainable or impossible. You may even get butterflies in your stomach when you decide to run the rapids, take an acting class or even go camping alone in a foreign country.

After marriage, I never gave much thought to *creating* a life for myself; I just concentrated on ways to live the one I had. Sure, I had fantasies—an exciting career, a dynamite wardrobe, a gorgeous home with the "perfect family," money, success, travel, losing that infamous last ten pounds so I would *finally* have my longed-for, thin body. But in reality, my young adulthood was overshadowed by my constant struggle to cope with a seemingly perpetual wave of problems as they came at me, and striving to make ends meet.

Then, after my divorce, I found myself falling prey to the empty nest syndrome, agonizing over loneliness and dwelling on thoughts of becoming decrepit and undesirable.

There was no doubt about it; I was in the throes of a full-scale conflict. Either I took charge and conquered aging or it would conquer me. As far as I could see, I had no choice. Nothing short of a miracle would do the trick. I would have to completely transform my life. I analyzed what steps I would have to take to accomplish this.

First, I made a decision: I had better learn to stop suffering and love aging since there was no avoiding it. As an added incentive, I also told myself that if I conquered my own aging I could give my children, and the world, a living example of a mature woman who became more and more vibrant with the passage of time. With this exciting challenge igniting my spirit, I began a search for a new, fulfilling life.

My first step was to sit down and actually define my desires and needs. Then I began to travel; I made new friends; I experimented boldly and beautifully.

Then I starting Blitzing—getting rid of possessions, memories, ideas, even relationships—things that were trapping me in the past. The results have been astounding. Bravely striking out, I lived on a Caribbean island—Tortola, in the British Virgin Islands—for two years, flying back and forth to New York and California every time I needed a shot of civilization and cash. I swam, scuba dived, danced and sailed. I meditated for hours, sunned naked on secluded beaches. I came to know myself in the deepest sense.

With this newfound sense of who I am, I am finally able to live the life I always dreamed of living. I now have a life of excitement, adventure and the knowledge that I truly make a difference in this world.

In your final written exercise, Getting the Life I Love, you will define *exactly* what you want from life. You might find out that you have been stingy with yourself, withholding your warmth, feelings or true beauty. You may decide, as I did, to give more of yourself in order to achieve this wonderful life. You will take those dreams that have been floating around in your head for as long as you can remember and write them down as specifically as you would the agenda for a business meeting or plans for a trip. When doing this exercise, make sure that you use words that inspire and empower you to take action, for in action lies ultimate fulfillment.

Even though your goals seem impossible, or you don't know how you'll accomplish them, keep focusing on them as if they are already achieved. Visualize and sense your goals until you get a taste of how it feels to be living them. Make your statements positive and powerful, without a subtext of "this could never be" or even "someday . . . if only." Savor the sensations now.

To give your goals an even bigger boost, provide yourself with a time line. Decide when you will complete a task or perform an activity. This time factor is not a drop-dead deadline, like income tax day, but is instead a target for you to work toward.

If you still need more proof of the power of dreams, consider this very book that you are now reading. Who would have thought that little, curly-haired Hattie Messner from Brooklyn would be telling people how to do *anything*, much less entering beauty contests, appearing on television, giving lectures around the world, patenting two chairs—and writing this book?

As to *my* future, here goes:

I will open five international RetroAge Spas by the year 2001, the first on an island in the Caribbean. One of my tropical spas will be devoted to healthy families. I envision babies birthed in clear, warm water, and mothers and fathers receiving exquisite care along with their newborns. Futhermore, each spa will support local organic farming, humane treatment of animals and clean water and air.

And I'll appear in an unretouched nude spread in *Playboy*.

And I'll star in a singing-dancing-comedy celebration of life at Radio City Music Hall.

And I'll host *Saturday Night Live*.

And I'll see the verb RetroAge become part of the English language.

And my anti-aging chair design will be incorporated into offices, cars and airlines.

And . . . Now, get this: I even let my mind conjure up a satellite spa in outer space. The Spaship RetroAge?

Granted, my dreams may appear wildly far-fetched to you, but there they are in black and white. Ready to happen.

I invite and encourage you to let your fantasies soar. Perhaps we won't reach all our goals. Perhaps they'll even be surpassed! Actually, in some way, it doesn't really matter. Our dreams keep us awake.

So get to work!

GETTING THE LIFE I LOVE

A word of caution: Do *not* let your Negative Aging Voice with its resignation and cynicism sabotage this process. Resist censoring yourself. No fantasy is taboo. Follow your deepest, most pleasurable images rather than those that conjure up strife, toil, doom and gloom. You never know where your dreams will take you.

Let your imagination soar as you fill in the blanks of this chart. Remember the Hattitude: Impossible = I'm Possible! Your future is truly in your hands.

What I Want That I Haven't Been Getting	What I Will Do About It and By When

Now go back over your list and arrange your new goals in chronological order: What you plan to accomplish in one month, six months, one year, five years, ten years, etc.

The very act of writing these dream-based goals as graphically and specifically as you can is the catalyst that helps make them happen. You will find that the more vividly you visualize the results, the more effective you become in creating your own life.

YES, it takes courage and self-discipline.

YES, it is hard work.

But most important:

YES, you can create yourself as truly ageless.

For me, RetroAging has extended my life far beyond the border of my self. Having accomplished my goals for anti-aging, I was left with a surprising void: I had this great life now, but what would—or could—I do with it in the future? I decided to dedicate myself to transforming the world's ideas about aging. I believe that accepting and loving ourselves through the aging process is crucial to the survival of our planet.

That's quite a sweeping statement: *Survival of our planet.*

Let me explain how I made this connection. It is easy for us to love what's exquisite, beautiful and perfect. Our task, as individuals and as a society, is to love ourselves and our universe even when it isn't these things. As we develop that deep, internal respect for ourselves, the universe will shift.

It might be valuable to consider some facts surrounding feelings we have about our bodies. For instance, the most beautiful, physically privileged individuals pick and peck at themselves, even at the apex of their pulchritude. It's the hair, or the nose, or the shape, size or location of the breasts. We're too tall or too short, too thin or too thick; but always that self-condemnation. Now, if this appears in the most beautiful people, multiply it a thousandfold for the remainder of us mortals, most of whom look to these self-deprecating beauties with jealous admiration. As you see, there are a vast number of human beings involved in serious self-contempt on this planet.

For many of us, negative self-image starts in childhood and escalates as we grow. It begins with nuggets of disapproval and fear that we receive from our parents, teachers and ultimately from society. We suffer from an epidemic of self-hatred, with aging a prime target of this malice. We all are bound by the same life forces. Like the tides, we rise and fall. We were no happier then than now . . . nor are we happier now than then. In truth, there is little difference between being young and being old: Life is magnificent, and monstrous, at various turns. But as humans we keep searching for the reasons for our sadnesses and our fears. As we get older, it is easy to place the blame on aging.

How much more difficult is it for us to keep loving ourselves, for instance, as we see our flesh sag, our skin become crepey and our energy wane? Much more. We fear that we must give up the joys of running down the beach or making ardent love. Then we resent and bemoan the fact that our less-than-young bodies won't perform *exactly* as they did when we were children. What we have lost sight of is the fact that our bodies, though they are constantly changing, *do* have the capacity to move fully and freely at any age.

It's all about perception. Some days, when I look into my mirror, I see a wrinkled, old face, and other days, I see a cute, open-eyed, curly-haired child. They are both me. So when you see yourself looking dreadful, don't believe that aging has turned you irreversibly into an old person. Think about what you are feeling, what messages you are listening to. And then turn those negative messages around and watch the image in the mirror change.

Self-love makes miracles possible.

Children don't even see what we adults perceive as flaws. They just see their granny and they love her. She has white hair and her arms wiggle. They're fun to play with. And Grandpa—he has a big belly that jiggles when he walks. Uncle Joe has teeth that fall down when you push his nose.

We must cultivate the openness and curiosity, the truthful gaze of a child, devoid of judgment and evaluations that cause us to hate ourselves and others. We can learn to be playful about our own imperfections as well as those of others.

This child's vision gives us true eternal youth, for as you *see*, so shall you *be*. How wonderful for us to have the chance to turn about that life-denying vision and create a loving, caring, life-affirming attitude. You won't develop this skill overnight. A reminder: It took years to cultivate that negative self-image. Give yourself time for this new way of being to flower. One of the blessings of aging, for me, is that it has given me time to learn to love myself, to develop self-respect and the knowledge that I can trust myself to be a responsible, caring human being.

I often muse about how long it took me to become whole and healthy. Wouldn't it be a shame if I didn't have the stamina to enjoy my hard-earned sanity? Fortunately, RetroAge has given me the means to achieve lifelong youth and I fully intend to enjoy it well into my eighties . . . nineties . . . who knows?

As you open yourself to the possibility of growing younger year after year, you will meet more and more people on this wondrous path. They will welcome and help you, and you, in turn, will welcome and help others. We humans have that opportunity. It can create our glory . . . or our doom.

The choice is ours.

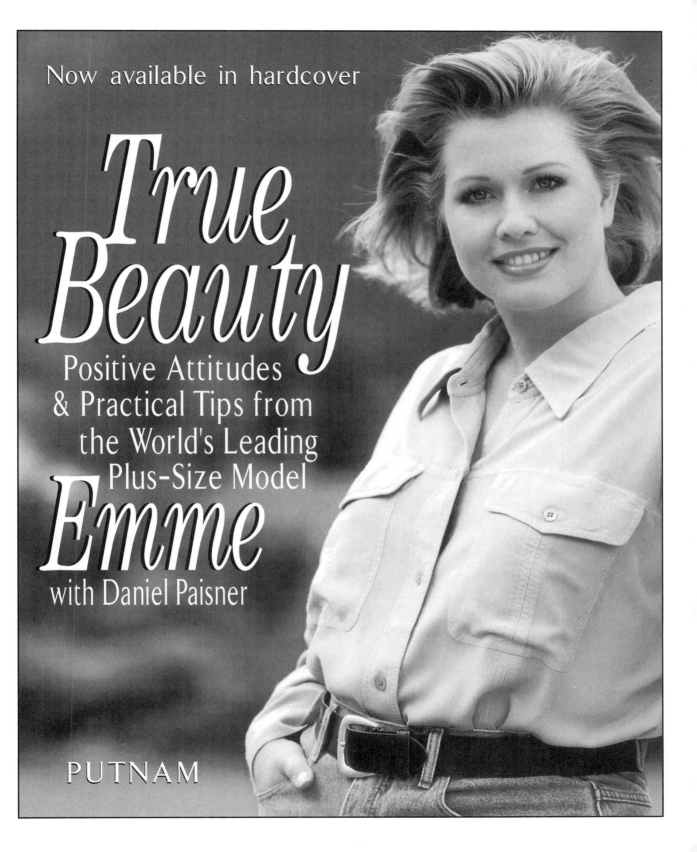